Syphilis

Syphilis

Medicine, Metaphor, and Religious Conflict in Early Modern France

Deborah N. Losse

THE OHIO STATE UNIVERSITY PRESS • COLUMBUS

Copyright © 2015 by The Ohio State University.
All rights reserved.

Library of Congress Cataloging-in-Publication Data
Losse, Deborah N., 1944– , author.
  Syphilis : medicine, metaphor, and religious conflict in early modern France / Deborah N. Losse.
     p. ; cm.
  Includes bibliographical references and index.
  ISBN 978-0-8142-1272-1 (hardback : alk. paper) — ISBN 978-0-8142-9377-5 (cd-rom)
  I. Title.
  [DNLM: 1. Medicine in Literature—France. 2. Syphilis—history—France. 3. History, Early Modern 1451–1600—France. 4. Religion and Medicine—France. WC 11 GF7]
  RC201.6.F8
  616.95'130094409031—dc23
                              2014033909

Cover design by AuthorSupport.com
Text design by Juliet Williams
Type set in Adobe Sabon

♾ The paper used in this publication meets the minimum requirements of the American National Standard for Information Sciences—Permanence of Paper for Printed Library Materials. ANSI Z39.48–1992.

9 8 7 6 5 4 3 2 1

CONTENTS

Preface and Acknowledgments vii

INTRODUCTION 1

1 Rabelais, the Codpiece, and Syphilis 11

2 Erasmus, *The Colloquies,* and Syphilis 30

3 Cannibalism and Syphilis in the Context of Religious Controversy 46

4 Wild Appetites/Appétit[s] Desordonné[s]: Cannibalism, Siege, and the Sins of the Old World in Jean de Léry 66

5 The Old World Meets the New in Montaigne's *Essais*: Syphilis, Cannibalism, and Empirical Medicine 85

6 Tragic Afflictions: D'Aubigné's *Tragiques* 106

CONCLUSION 121

Notes 129
Bibliography 155
Index 161

PREFACE *and* ACKNOWLEDGMENTS

THE TOPIC of this study grew out of an invitation from Philippe Desan, editor of *Montaigne Studies,* to return to a subject on which I had written earlier, Montaigne and the New World, and to contribute an article to a forthcoming volume on *Montaigne et le nouveau monde* XX, 1–2 (2010). In the course of research, it became apparent to me that Montaigne's fascination with cannibalism, the inhabitants of the New World, and those inhabitants' cultural practices was linked to his interest in the plants and remedies that were being imported to the Old World. Guaiacum was a case in point, a South American plant from which the indigenous inhabitants of the New World and the physicians and surgeons of the Old World prepared decoctions judged helpful in the treatment of the pox. Montaigne's interest in the exotic plants brought back from the New World is set within a negative context of the cachet that exotic provenance and expense brings to remedies: "Si les nations desquelles nous retirons le gayac, la salseperille et le bois desquine, ont des medecins, combien pensons nous, par cette mesme recommendation de l'estrangeté, la rareté et la cherté, qu'ils facent feste de nos choux et de nostre persil: car qui oseroit mespriser les choses recherchées de si loing, au hasard d'une si longue peregrination et si perilleuse?" (II: 37, 772A/585–86) [If the countries from which we get guaiacum, sarsaparilla, and chinaroot have doctors, how much, we may imagine, through this same recommendation of strangeness, rarity, and costliness, must they prize our cabbages and our parsley! For who would dare despise things sought out at a distance, at the risk of such a long and perilous voyage?][1] The essayist goes on to attack the sudden changes in treatment that trouble the habits and routines of the patients. He singles out his contemporary physicians Paracelsus, Fioravanti, and Argenterius for criticism: "Car ils ne changent pas seulement une recepte, mais, à ce qu'on me dict, toute la contexture et police du corps de la medicine" (II: 37, 772A/586) [For they change not merely one prescription, but, so they tell me, the whole contexture and order of the study of medicine].

Fioravanti attracted clients with his drastic and controversial treatments for syphilis but remained a strong advocate for the efficacy of guaiacum for his patients suffering from the pox. The above passage from Montaigne and his further adoption of sickness, including syphilis, as a metaphor for what was ailing France at the time of the civil and religious conflicts during the Wars of Religion encouraged me to look at other authors living in sixteenth-century France. How widespread was the confluence of the topics of cannibalism, syphilis, and the ravages of the Wars of Religion? It will become obvious from the chapters to follow that the spread of the pox from the New World to the Old, following the return of the men who had accompanied Columbus to the Americas, had seized the imagination of the inhabitants of Europe because they witnessed the spread of the disease as well as the destruction it brought to the family and social structures.

Many people have helped to advance this project. First, Arizona State University, the provost Elizabeth D. Phillips, the president Michael M. Crow, and former vice president and dean of the College of Liberal Arts and Sciences Quentin Wheeler were generous in allowing me to take a research leave from my administrative position to travel to Paris to work at the Bibliothèque Nationale de France (BnF). Special thanks to Linda C. Lederman and Sid P. Bacon for their encouragement and counsel, precious in that Sid did not live long after and yet had so much wisdom to offer his friends, colleagues, and family. I would like to thank the director of the School of International Letters and Cultures, Robert Joe Cutter, and my colleagues in French and Italian for their support. As always, I appreciate the kindness and support of my family, John, Kate, and Owen. Finally, I wish to thank Philippe Desan, editor of *Montaigne Studies,* for kind permission to reprint portions of "The Old World Meets the New in Montaigne's *Essais:* The Nexus of Syphilis, Cannibalism, and Empirical Medicine," *Montaigne Studies* 22, 1–2 (2010): 85–99.

INTRODUCTION

HE FRANCISCAN cosmographer André Thevet was indeed prescient when he conjectured that the "maladie de pians" in Brazil was none other than the pox ("la belle vérole") that had spread so rapidly throughout Christianity ("toute la Chrestienté"). He added that it was an illness common to all humans ("un mal commun de tout le monde") and not originating in Naples or in France, as the nomenclature "mal de Naples" or "morbus gallicus" would suggest. There was ample blame for its spread, although Thevet speculated that it had its roots with those who engaged in relations with the hot-blooded indigenous women ("ces femmes ainsy eschauffees") of the New World.[1] Lewd behavior ("paillardise") was at its roots, and neither the population of the New World nor of Europe was exempt of responsibility. What the cosmographer understood on his sojourn in Brazil was that what he called the pox, and what he and his fellow Frenchman Jean de Léry heard the Tupinamba call "pians," was related to the vicious outbreak of the pox or "grosse vérole" in Europe.[2]

A modern scholar, Francesco Guerra, states that the various strains of what we now call syphilis—*pinta* (found in America), yaws (found in central Africa and the East and West Indies), endemic syphilis (seen in Africa, Arabia, Siberia, and central Australia), and venereal syphilis (common to urban areas)—"are morphologically indistinguishable."[3] That a Franciscan (Thevet) and a Huguenot (Léry) should agree in describing a sexually transmitted disease observed among the Tupinamba in Brazil and yet write competing versions of New World exploration from opposite sides of the religious conflict waging in France speaks to the centrality of the spread of syphilis and to its hold on the French mind. The disease threatened the health of the body, the institution of marriage and the family, as well as the survival of humanity. The Wars of Religion menaced the body politic, civil institutions, and the law. The dual threat—to the individual and to society—moved some of the greatest writers of France and Europe in the sixteenth century, including Erasmus, Rabelais, Montaigne, and Agrippa d'Aubigné, as well as many poets, to view the pox as a metaphor for civic and religious disorder in Europe.

Between the outbreak of syphilis, shortly after the return of Columbus's men to Europe and the commencement of violence that would characterize the French Wars of Religion, a third element appeared that mediated the link between the first two phenomena. The chroniclers of the New World exploration became increasingly intrigued with the topic of cannibalism. The failure of the indigenous people of the New World to respect the division of species into natural categories, thereby falling into the error of ingesting their own species as food, was proof to many New World chroniclers that these same people lacked the power to reason. As Anthony Pagden states, "Like the two sexual crimes—sodomy and bestiality—of which the Indians were also accused . . . their cannibalism demonstrated that they could not clearly distinguish between the rigid and self-defining categories into which the natural world was divided."[4]

In Italy, the controversial surgeon, Leonardo Fioravanti, famed for his unorthodox treatment of victims of syphilis, blamed the outbreak of syphilis on acts of cannibalism when the army cooks in Naples created stews out of human limbs to feed the soldiers. This "unnatural" behavior produced the disease, which then could only be treated by the "expulsion of the same bodily corruption."[5] Sickness, as Eamon states, carried for Fioravanti "moral overtones" as well as physiological symptoms, and for him, the acts of cannibalism at the siege of Naples revealed the bodily and moral laxity exhibited by the butchers and cooks who deceived the soldiers into consuming human flesh (Eamon, 16, 21). Unlike most of his contemporary medical practitioners, chroniclers, and thinkers, he blamed the Europeans for the onset of syphilis in Europe (Eamon, 22). The violent purge, for which Fioravanti was known and criticized, was the only way to purify the body and ease the patient's suffering. Hence syphilis and cannibalism were inextricably intertwined in the Renaissance mind. In chapters 3 and 4 I will show how cannibalism and syphilis were linked by such chroniclers as Thevet and Léry.

I have briefly alluded to the names by which syphilis was known in the late fifteenth and sixteenth centuries. In her translation and commentary of Girolamo Fracastoro's *Syphilis sive morbus gallicus,* from which in later centuries the disease took its name, after the rebellious shepherd Syphilus, Jacqueline Vons states that in a Europe ravaged by foreign wars, it is not surprising to find a new disease attributed to the other—to foreigners. To the Italian Fracastoro (1476/78?–1553), faced with the invasion of the armies of the French king Charles VIII, it was the *morbus gallicus;* for the German-speaking Joseph Grünpeck (1473–1532), it was the *mala de Franzos.* In writing up his treatment for the disease in 1541, Remacle Fuchs (1510–87) acknowledged three names: *Morbi* Hispanici *quem allii* Gallicum, *alii* Neapolitanicum *appellant,* thus making the Spanish, the French, and the people of Naples responsible for the disease (Fracastor, XIX). Vons also mentions William Cowes shifting the title of his work *A New and Approved Treatise Concerning the Cure of the French Pockes By the Unctions* (1575) to *A Briefe and Necessarie Treatise, Touching the Cure of the Disease Now Usually Called Lues Venerea* (1596), a change that reflects the Latin name by which the disease had become known (Fracastor, XIX). While the term *morbus neapolitanus* was less common, the name indicates that the people took notice that the spread of the disease coincided with the arrival of French and mercenary soldiers in Naples in February 1495 (Fracastor, XX). One appellation for the disease, *gorre des marranes*, reflects a tendency to stigmatize an entire community, in this case, the Jews who migrated from Spain to France upon their forced conversion to Catholicism.[6] Apart from names denoting a foreign origin of the disease, the term *lues venerea,* connecting the pollution or filth (*lues*) to Venus and the sexual act, predominated among Latinist physicians, while the name *grosse vérole* or *grande vérole* prevailed in the French vernacular writing.[7]

I have talked about the onset of syphilis and the link to cannibalism, but before proceeding onwards, let me address the chronology of the French Wars of Religion in which the rhetoric of pox and cannibalism unfolds. The period of religious controversy that spans this book begins with the early years of evangelical humanism at the outset of the sixteenth century. The influence of Guillaume Briçonnet (1472–1536) on Marguerite de Navarre, at the time Duchess of Alençon, and by extension on her brother François I, has been documented by Henry Heller and, later, by Ehsan Ahmed.[8] Briçonnet's correspondence with Marguerite between early June 1521 and November 18, 1524, critiques human reason and praises the life that gives itself to the spirit ("esperit vivifiant")—the Word of Christ ("la semence du Verbe superceleste").[9] It is through the spirit, not reason, that humans can grasp the Word (Ahmed, 616). Briçonnet's critique of human reason aims at the Faculty of Theology of Paris, who used reason to attack subversive texts such as the writings of Jacques Lefèvre d'Étaples, and "seeks to persuade not only Marguerite but also François I and their mother Louise de Savoie to pursue 'la restitucion and reformacion de son [i.e., Jesus'] Eglise'" (Briçonnet et Marguerite d'Angoulème, I: 166; Ahmed, 617). This early evangelism, giving primacy to the spirit over reason, informs the works of both François Rabelais and Erasmus, the subjects of chapter 1 and 2 of this book.

Denis Crouzet observes that the early progression of reform, built on the exchange of ideas across Europe, brought a rather slow progression of new doctrine. He points out François I's hesitation, when his sister Marguerite was corresponding with Briçonnet, and Briçonnet's hope that the spirit will work through the royal family to preserve the church, then plagued by "orgoeul, lascivitté et avarice" (Briçonnet and Marguerite de Navarre, I: 166; Ahmed, 617).[10] With the placing of statements printed in Neuchâtel opposing the Mass, François I perceived the danger that the reform doctrine posed for the stability of the monarchy. Crouzet remarks that not only did the king engage in a very public eucharistic procession with his children, but six heretics were burned during the rite ("six hérétiques sont brûlés"; 19). In 1540, the Edict of Fontainebleau empowered the *parlements* to oversee accusations of heresy.[11] Henri II continued the persecution of the Protestant heretics, with 500 heretics sentenced between 1549 and 1551 by the Chambre ardente, a special court set up within the Parlement de Paris (Knecht, 3).

As the number of Calvinist missions grew, so did the number of violent incidents against Calvinists. Yet the Huguenots also began to engage in political intrigue, as evidenced by the Huguenot La Renaudie's involvement in the Conspiracy of Amboise in 1560 to replace the young king François II with a regent of the reformist Bourbon family. This plot was not supported by Calvin nor by many Huguenot churches and so did not succeed (Knecht, 9).

Rather than being followed by a period of recrimination against the Huguenots, there was a general pardon, known as the Edict of Amboise (1560). All Huguenots except the conspirators were pardoned, providing that they returned to the Catholic faith. With the death of the François II in the same year, Catherine de Medici became regent. In her desire to restore order and to ease tension between Catholics and Protestants, she convoked the Colloquy of Poissy, where basic differences regarding the Eucharist only intensified disagreements. Were the sacraments the real body and blood of Christ or symbolic of the same? The *parlement* deputies gathered at Saint-Germain crafted the Edict of Saint-Germain or the Edict of Janvier (January 17, 1562), permitting the Huguenots freedom to worship in the countryside but not in the cities. The ire of the Catholics at this nod toward freedom of conscience—freedom to worship as one wills—propelled the long period of violence that would last until the Edict of Nantes in 1598. A series of eight wars of religion weakened the French state, decimated the people, and threatened the monarchy itself (Knecht, 30–33; Crouzet, 24–25).[12] All pretense at mediation and reconciliation came to an end at the Massacre of Vassy in March 1562, when the troops of François, Duke of Guise, attacked a group of Huguenots who were exercising their right to worship as set out in the Edict of Janvier.

The selection of works to be examined in this book reflects what was happening on the political and religious front. The rhetoric of paradox, wordplay, and parody found in the works of Erasmus, Rabelais, and Du Fail gave way to a more aggressive language of attack aimed against Catholics by Léry, Théodore de Bèze, or Agrippa d'Aubigné or against Protestants by Artus Désiré and Pierre de Ronsard in the second half of the sixteenth century. Montaigne would denounce the abuses on both sides. The literary timeline follows roughly the period of intensifying violence in the political and religious spheres. As for the chronology of the pandemic, I follow the slow and steady rise in the earliest years of the outbreak of the pox, followed by the increasing virulence between 1515 and 1540 and the gradual steadying of outbreaks and recognition that the cases were not quite as intense in the years 1550 to 1600. Francisco López de Gómara confirmed the reduction in vigor and violence of the disease around mid-century when he published his *Historia general de las Indias* (1553).[13]

The topic of syphilis spans literary genres. Because of the attention Rabelais paid to his "goutteux" (gouty) and "verolez" (poxied), one might think that syphilis was the unique purview of satirical narrative, the subject of chapter 1. As I shall show in chapter 2, Erasmus devoted several colloquies to exploring the impact of syphilis on social institutions, particularly on the institution of marriage and the family. Chapter 3 explores how satirical verse attributes licentious behavior and the consequent physical deformities brought on by syphilis to both Catholic and Protestant clergy. Travel literature written by the cosmographer Thevet and the ethnographer Léry explores the conjunction of cannibalism and syphilis among the Tupi people. Siege literature, whether in the form of memoirs, such as Léry's *Histoire mémorable du siège de Sancerre,* or in poetic form, such as d'Aubigné's *Les Tragiques,* weaves the threads of cannibalism and wanton behavior into a tapestry of lapsed morals that threatened French society in the time of the wars of religion. The first work is discussed in chapter 4 and was written immediately after the collapse of Sancerre, when it was besieged by the royal armies. The second work, the subject of chapter 6, was the result of d'Aubigné's long reflection on the suffering caused by Catholic extremists to the Huguenots, but the author is clear that it is the kingdom of France, its people, and its institutions that have suffered insurmountable damage. This view was shared by Ronsard and Montaigne as well and reflected the growing violence and disrespect for the law.

While siege literature seems inspired by the need to bear witness to human suffering, so in fact is the essay, as will be evident in chapter 5 of this book. Montaigne expanded the scope of the essay to bear witness to his family's flight from his estate during an outbreak of the plague as well as an outbreak in violence in nearby Castillon. These events, along with personal encounters with Catholic and Protestant forces in and around Montaigne, led the essayist to depart from the more succinct form of the essay that had characterized the first and parts of the second book of his *Essais* to return with increasing regularity to self-portraiture. It is in the context of discussing how children resemble parents that he brings up medicine, referring to the family-inherited ailment, kidney stones, and the family distrust of the practice of medicine. From there, he associates the exotic remedies brought back from the New World, such as guaiac for the treatment of syphilis, with the names of the medical practitioners who espouse extreme and novel cures along with the use of such rare plants: Paracelsus, Fioravanti, and Argentier ("Paracelse, Fioravanti et Argenterius").[14] For Montaigne, this was all at the expense of the "pauvre patient" (the long-suffering patient), for whom such violent purgatives only increased pain and suffering. The new form he developed—the essay—was the latest genre to apply medical analogies to the civil disorder and religious conflicts occurring in France.

The two phenomena, the epidemic of syphilis in the Old World and the violent religious and civil strife, converged as the physical patients in Europe gave way to a metaphorical patient—France itself, ravaged by competing factions: Catholics, Huguenots, and the extreme Catholic party known as the *Ligue*. Montaigne would refer to "nostre mort publique, ses symptomes et sa forme" (III: 12, 1046/800) [our public death, its symptoms and its form]. D'Aubigné describes France as "une mère affligée": "Je veux peindre la France une mere affligée" [I want to paint France as an suffering mother].[15] She is bloodied by her two sons, Esau (Catholics) and Jacob (Protestants), fighting over her breasts, and leaving only blood instead of milk to feed them. She grieves: "Je n'ay plus que du sang pour vostre nourriture" (*Les Tragiques*, I: 269, v. 130) [I have only blood for your food]. Physical decline becomes a moral decline; an individual illness gives way to a moribund body politic no longer able to defend itself from internal and external threats.

The fact that writers and thinkers in the sixteenth century should view a protracted civil conflict as a prolonged outbreak of a new disease should not surprise those familiar with Renaissance thought. Michel Foucault reminds us that until the end of the sixteenth century, resemblance or likeness played a foundational role in the ways humanist thinkers, writers, and artists acquired knowledge: "Jusqu'à la fin du XVIe siècle, la ressemblance a joué un rôle bâtisseur dans le savoir de la culture occiedentale."[16] New phenomena were observed and compared to objects with which the observer was familiar. With simile, the two phenomena compared are tied in space and time when the two are evoked together vocally, in writing, or in a painting. Metaphor, what Foucault terms emulation or *aemulatio*, is likeness freed from spatial propinquity and spatial law, "une sorte de convenance, mais qui serait affranchie de la loi du lieu" (Foucault, 34). What we see as metaphor suggests rather than states, and as Foucault remarks, is akin to the play between mirror and reflection (34).[17]

So, when Montaigne mentions epidemics or common diseases ("maladies populaires") to refer to religious conflicts raging in France, and indeed outside his very estate, he is referring not to a physical illness as much as to violence and fighting among the French people: "En ces maladies populaires, on peut distinguer sur le commencement les sains des malades; mais quand elles viennent à durer, comme la nostre, tout le corps s'en sent" (III: 12, 1041B/796) [In these epidemics one can distinguish at the beginning the well from the sick; but when they come to last, like ours, the whole body is affected]. It is clear he is referring to armed conflict as an illness or epidemic because he goes on to rail against mercenaries or "borrowed soldiers" ("soldats empruntez"; 1042B/7960). He suggests the likeness between epidemic and civil war by enumerating the effects—the infected, stinking body—common to the sickroom and to the battlefield. Joel Fineman reminds us that describing "political, military, and social facts" in medical terms goes all the way back to Thucydides, who adopted the "semiological language and method of the Hippocratic doctor": "diagnosis," "prognosis," and "natural cause" or "*prophasis.*"[18] Like Montaigne, d'Aubigné refers to war-torn France as a patient. In a letter to Marie de Medici, the poet speaks of the necessity of entering into the sick room ("entrer dans la chambre") with a vial of medicine in hand ("avec la fiole à la main").[19]

The somewhat hidden nature of the metaphor, a figure that, as Hayden White tells us, "gives direction for finding the set of images that are intended to be associated with the thing," has advantages in the incendiary atmosphere of Paris in the wake of the Saint Bartholomew Massacre.[20] Sometimes, the pox and the lascivious behavior with which it was associated served both Protestants and Catholics as a means to attack the opposition without engaging in the more risky language of theology. At other times, theology and medicine overlap, as will be seen in the discussion of the work of Léry, where lechery, theology, and cannibalism are intertwined. The metaphor chosen by the historian or poet becomes a way in which the author presents the world and orders the facts (White, 47). For White, the images, in this case the metaphors of cannibalism and syphilis, "provide a system of translation which allows the viewer to link the image [here cannibalism or syphilis] with the thing represented," the Eucharist or the French Wars of Religion (White, 47).

Beyond the metaphors in which cannibalism points toward the substantive difference between the Catholic and Protestant views of the Host, or in which the metaphor of syphilis is broadened to point to wider corruption in the social fabric, another metaphor, much used in the sermons of Saint Augustine, is that of the "Christus Medicus," an image that was popular in the writings and iconography of Renaissance Europe. John Henderson mentions the use of the image of Christ touching the wound in his side placed prominently in the lunette leading to the cemetery of Florence's main hospital, Santa Maria Nuova. He notes that the positioning of the figure of Man of Sorrows, as this figure was called, represents "a door to salvation."[21] Rudolph Arbesmann tells us that Saint Augustine returned again and again in his sermons to the healing image of Christ, who through a humble action took the form of man to redeem the sins of humankind. Healer of soul and body, unlike earthly physicians, he is the model of humility.[22]

New epidemics demand new spiritual tools for easing the corporal and spiritual suffering of the indisposed. Christ's wounded body, with his hand in the wound, reminds the faithful that through their pain and suffering, they may find redemption. Like the "verollez" of the "Patenostre des Verollez," those who are exiled, starved, and mutilated may find that God "gard(e) place en Paradis" to deliver them at last from the earthly suffering they have endured.[23] Faced with the rapid spread of the pox, along with periods of plague, the hospitals were crowded; new types of hospitals were established to deal with the *incurabili*—sufferers from the strange and virulent new disease (Henderson, 71). Physicians such as François Rabelais returned to the Augustinian image—Rabelais in the prologue to his *Quart Livre,* as he ponders the suffering of the "goutteux" and "verollez."[24]

That the chronicles describing cannibalism and the occurrence of syphilis in the New World should happen at the very time of the outbreak of violence between Catholics and Protestants fed the rhetoric of the pamphlets distributed by both sides. The Catholic concept of transubstantiation, as the Huguenot Léry states, comes very close to cannibalism: "Ils vouloyent neantmoins non seulement grossierement, plustost que spirituellement, manger la chair de Jesus-Christ, mais qui pis estoit, à la manière des sauvages nommez *Ou-ëtacas* . . . , ils vouloyent mascher et avaler toute crue" [Nevertheless they wanted not only to eat the flesh of Jesus Christ grossly rather than spiritually, but what was worse, like the savages named Ouetaca . . . , they wanted to chew and swallow it raw].[25] A Protestant satirical poem, *Satyres chrestiennes de la cuisine papale,* attributed by some to Théodore de Bèze, refers to the Catholics as "Anthropophages" and "Theophages" ("Man-eaters" and "God-eaters").[26] The Catholic Artus Désiré throws accusations of lust and wantonness at his Protestant counterparts, calling them "charnelz" and "lubriques." In his verse their heresy is transformed into a stinking, putrid infection—not unlike the open pustules of syphilis: "puante"/"fluante"/"infection."[27] The common insult on both sides is wantonness or "paillardise." While not engaging in the rhetoric of the pox in his rebukes against Protestant acts of sedition and self-serving interpretations of the gospels, Ronsard gives a strong rebuttal to the accusation that he himself was infected with the disease. In "Response de Pierre de Ronsard aux injures et calomnies de je ne sçay quels predicanteraux et ministreaux de Genéve," he turns the accusations of the Huguenots against themselves as he shows just who is likely to spread both the pox and injustice through the kingdom of France.[28]

The language of cannibalism and medicine infuses the religious debate and inflames the open sores of civic conflict. It will be clear throughout this book that writers from Erasmus to d'Aubigné spoke of violence in Europe—whether caused by national rivalries or religious differences—as a danger to the health and well-being of the continent and its peoples. Violence is often framed in terms of an illness; the state subsumes the individual. Restoring the state and the continent to good health should be the aim of all people. Erasmus's butcher in his colloquy "A Fish Diet" speaks of healing the sores of conflict between Charles V and François I rather than simply applying a topical remedy that merely conceals them.[29] As Marjorie O'Rourke Boyle observes, Erasmus viewed the republic as a kind of body subject to illness: "The republic is a kind of body, . . . Its pestilence and disease are evil mores."[30] D'Aubigné makes a similar analogy when he writes to the young Duke of Montmorency: "Le royaume est malade de la subversion de toutes choses."[31] In another letter, this time to the Queen Mother, Marie de Medici, he likens France's illness to an internal or implicit illness in which a remedy to one member creates open sores in another member.[32]

As I advance in the analysis of the works of some key writers of prose, poetry, chronicles, and essays in the sixteenth century, it will become obvious that from the beginning, conflict between nations or within a single nation was viewed as hazardous to the health of the states involved. A kingdom reflected the health and welfare of its people—when one suffered, the health of the whole was at risk. The outbreak of syphilis at the end of the fifteenth century, causing a pandemic that struck terror into the hearts of all, seized the imagination of all Europeans and led them to extend the images of cruel and excruciating suffering to the body politic, opened up and ripped apart by interpersonal conflict caused by religious differences, overriding personal ambition, and prejudice. Erasmus, Rabelais, and Montaigne adopted the analogy between the health of the individual and the health of the nation in order to mediate the growing political and religious conflict.[33] This should not be surprising given their belief in moderation as a remedy for most things. What should be astonishing is that even the most partisan writers understood that just as surely as syphilis—the unintended consequence of New World expansion—had ravaged the population of Europe, so too external and internal rivalry based on religious differences and personal ambition had destroyed the state's ability to prosper, to nourish its people, and to extend its cultural, scientific, and intellectual influence. Let me turn first to the works of François Rabelais to see how the virulence of the outbreak of syphilis had captivated the European imagination.

1

Rabelais, the Codpiece, and Syphilis

WHEN MIKHAIL BAKHTIN speaks of Rabelais's frequent evocation of the codpiece and of references to lovemaking, procreation, and venereal disease (his favored "vérolez" or "goutteux"), the Russian critic either does so in relation to the grotesque—the desire to show the body in "the act of becoming" (a body that "is never finished, never completed," one that "is continually built, created, builds and creates another body")—or in relation to the opposition between official or church culture and popular culture as represented by the marketplace and popular farce.[1] There is another reason, based in the history of the times, that explains why Rabelais would have given primacy to his "vérolez." Since the outbreak of syphilis in 1497, the cities of Europe were filled with patients who suffered the most visible ravages of the disease. From the time in which Rabelais embarked upon the publication of the tales of his giants Pantagruel and Gargantua in the period between 1532 and 1552, he had witnessed the spread of the pandemic across Europe. The French invasion of Italy served as a catalyst for the rapid growth of the disease from the returning sailors who had accompanied Columbus to the New World to the soldiers of Spanish, Italian, French, Swiss, and German origins who then returned to every corner in Europe to infect the inhabitants of their hometowns and cities: wives, wet nurses, babies, domestics, merchants, clergy, and nobility.[2] It was well known even in the sixteenth century that wet nurses and nursing mothers were at risk for passing the disease to the babies they nursed. No social class was exempt.[3] Evidence of the presence of "grosse vérole" or syphilis exists in Paris, Besançon, and Lyon in the edicts discovered by medical scholars of the disease, one being an Arrêt de Parlement de Paris dated as early as March 6, 1497, warning of the presence of persons suffering from the "grosse vérole" and of the dangers of contact with the diseased.[4]

Faced with the rapid spread of the *morbus gallicus* or the *mal français*, as it became known because of the coincidence of the presence of French soldiers in Italy at the time of the outbreak of the disease, Rabelais weaves the presence of those suffering from the disease throughout his work and gives them primacy by devoting his prologues to the "goutteux" and "vérolez"—those who enjoy life to the fullest through their drinking and sexual relations but also suffer the illnesses brought on by their sexual and gastronomical habits. As Bakhtin comments, gout and syphilis are in fact "joyeuses maladies" or happy diseases resulting from immoderate abuses of food and sexual pleasure (Bakhtin, 164/161). Such joyous flaunting of what Bakhtin calls the lower stratum or "bas corporel" is set in direct opposition to the drab hypocrisy and mournful demeanor of the priests and monks who spent more time fasting than attending to the needs of the poor. Jean Fernel, a contemporary of Rabelais and physician to Henri II and, by extension, to Diane de Poitiers, states very plainly that the disease is spread only through sexual intercourse or other impure contact ("il se contracte seulement par le coït ou par quelque autre impur").[5] While, as Bakhtin suggests, Rabelais may have been moved by the metaphorical interpretations of "la grosse vérole," the historic dimensions of the disease and the social changes in medical treatment, fashion, and social interaction caused by the ubiquitous presence of the disease is part of the fabric of Rabelais's work. What is of interest here is how his views of the disease, of its symptoms, treatment, and changes in dress necessitated by the disease, reflect ways in which the populace, physicians, artists, and writers dealt with the disease. Rabelais's evocation of syphilis goes well beyond what Bakhtin terms "la maladie à la mode" (Bakhtin, 164). As writer and physician, Rabelais probed the profound impact that the disease had on the way of life in the sixteenth century, and his work records this impact in ways that will be documented in this book.

If I begin with *Pantagruel*, first published in 1532, it is necessary to look only as far as the prologue, not yet dedicated to the "vérolez" but to the "Tresilllustres et Treschevaleureux champions" [Most illustrious and most valorous champions] to find a vivid portrait of the syphilitic covered in the therapeutic ointment that brought some relief and suffering from the symptoms brought on by the disease.[6]

> Mais que diray-je des pauvres vérolez et goutteux? O quantes foys nous les avons veu, à l'heure que ilz estoyent bien oingts et engressez à poinct, et le visaige leur reluysoit comme la claveure d'un charnier, et les dentz les tressailloyent comme font les marchettes d'un clavier d'orgues ou d'espinette quand on joue dessus et que le gosier leur escumoit comme à un verrat que les vaultres ont aculé entre les toilles! (*Pantagruel*, prologue, 215/134)

> But what am I to say of the poor poxies and gouties? How many times have we seen them, at the moment when they were well greased and duly anointed, as their face shone like the lock-plate of a larder, and their teeth were chattering like organ or spinet keys when someone plays on them, and their throat was frothing like a wild boar's that the dogs have run down into the toils!

The image of the ointment causing the syphilitic's face to shine would be taken up by other satirists, including in the *Satyres chrestiennes de la cuisine papale* (1560), whose author is widely believed to be Théodore de Bèze. The narrator describes "Nos Maistres sorbonniers / aussi luisans qu'une lanterne" [Our Sorbonne professors / As shiny as a lantern].[7] Chief among the "maistres sorbonniers" was a former president of the Parlement de Paris, *abbé* of Saint-Victor, and author of *Adversum pseudoevangelicam haeresim*, Pierre Lizet (1482–1554), mentioned later in the same work, who had banned many reform-minded theologians for heresy, including Bèze (*Satyres chrestiennes*, 160 n. 668).

Rabelais's description of the shiny, oily countenance of syphilitics, as well as those portraits by many of his contemporary writers, including Bèze and Erasmus, was accurate, as can be seen in the medications detailed in the works of physicians of the time. Writing one of the seminal works on syphilis, and the epic poem (*Syphilis sive morbus gallicus*), in which he links the name of the disease to the shepherd Syphile, doctor and poet Girolamo Fracastoro describes the ingredients that produced the oily appearance of the skin of those suffering from the pox. He recommends that should pernicious pain persist in gripping the body with convulsions, it could be calmed with an ointment made of mastic resin ("huile de mastic"), thick good fat ("la graisse d'oie bien épaisse"), and a mucilage made of various plant seeds, with liquid honey ("miel liquide") added.⁸ The plant seeds as well as saffron ("safran de Coryque") gave the ointment the orange or yellow color often mentioned by Renaissance writers. Fracastoro mentions, of course, the favored mercury ointment ("Argento melius persoluunt omnia vivo pars maior"; "Pour détruire complètement tous les signes du fléau, la majorité utilise avec plus de succès le vif-argent" [II: 48/49, vv. 270–71] [To completely destroy all the signs of the pestilence, most people use mercury to best effect]).

Rabelais's portrait of the suffering syphilitic, at once burning and teeth clacking, is reminiscent of Ulrich von Hutten's description of treatment for syphilis—a treatment he underwent and described with great precision. He observes the patient in an airless room ("une chambre en laquelle il ny aura guerre dair") in which a fire will be set in a chimney or, as in Germany, a stove ("en laquelle y ait tousiours un feu ou comme on fait en Germanie en une etuve").⁹ One can imagine that between the fever caused by the disease and the closed, hot room the patient would burn and shiver as fever and treatment rain their course, thus causing the alternation of red face and chattering teeth described by Rabelais. Ambroise Paré, king's surgeon to Henri II, Charles IX, and Henri III, prescribed an ointment of mercury mixed with lead and boiled in vinegar infused with sage, rosemary, thyme, and chamomile for relieving the discomfort of the open sores of syphilis.¹⁰ Such a treatment would produce the effects of Rabelais's "vérolez," "bien oingts et engressez à poinct," quoted above.

Immediately following his vivid description of his syphilitics, Rabelais observes that the anonymous popular chronicles of Gargantua serve to distract and console those suffering from the "grosse vérole," much as the *Life of Saint Margaret* ("la vie de la saincte Marguerite") does mothers in childbirth (*Pantagruel,* prologue, 215/134). This juxtaposition of a profane, popular work with a saint's life suggests a reform-minded Evangelical point of view poking fun at the importance of adoration of the saints in the everyday life of Christians. In fact, Jillings observes that the Protestant Hutten, in his *Febris I,* or *Fever I,* was perhaps the first, around 1520, to advance the disease metaphor as a religious polemic against the Catholic Church (Jillings, 1).¹¹ While Rabelais views his "vérolez" not as villains but as those who approach life with joy and gusto, his literary followers, whether Catholic or Protestant, would accuse their adversaries of lechery ("paillardise") and being the bearers of the pox which so threatened society's well-being. However, as can be seen in Rabelais's good-natured mention of the *Life of Saint Margaret,* his jest is not yet the embittered satire that would develop later see as the Wars of Religion reached their height.¹² Rabelais, after Hutten, would expand the metaphor connecting syphilis with religious polemic.

Panurge's proposal to build the walls of Paris out of the private parts of the women of Paris, lined up with the tallest women first, followed "par bonne symméterye d'architecture" progressively by the shorter women, occasions another reference to the likelihood that when the men approach the women to have sexual relations, an outbreak of the pox will follow: "Et puis, que les couillevrines se y vinsent froter, vous en verriez (par Dieu!) incontinent distiller de ce benoist fruict de grosse vérolle, menu comme pluye, sec au nom des diables!" (*Pantagruel*, ch. 15, 277/183) [And then if the culverins came and rubbed up against them, you would see (by God!) immediately distilled from them some of that blessed fruit of the pox, as fine as rain, dry in the devil's name!]. Not only is Rabelais building on the historic prevalence of the pox in Paris and on the steady rivalry between Charles V and François I, but he takes the occasion to pun on the usual means of defense—artillery in the form of *couleuvrines* and male reproductive organs, *couilles* to form the word *couillevrines*. Pox is seen here in its positive light—related to the lusty desires of the men to satisfy their needs. Panurge plays on Pantagruel's evocation of the Spartan Agesilaus's statement that the best protective walls of a city are the virtue and discipline of its citizen soldiers.¹³ In Panurge's version or inversion of the oft-quoted learned story, the virtue of the citizens is literally turned upside down in the "callibistrys des femmes" [women's watchamacallits]. The opposition of blessed fruit and pox ("benoist fruict" and "grosse vérolle) adds to the delightful juxtaposition of high and low culture, of abstinence and indulgence.

The pox enters through another strategy when Pantagruel invites Panurge to dress in his livery: "Vrayement, dist Pantagruel, tu es gentil compaignon; je te veux habiller de ma livrée" (*Pantagruel*, 15, 279/186) ["Really," said Pantagruel, "you're good company; I want to dress you in my livery"]. We don't generally think of Rabelais's works for their attention to changes in fashion. Yet, Panurge seeks a forward-looking style that is evolving:

> Et le feist vestir galantement selon la mode du temps qui couroit, *excepté que Panurge voulut que la braguette de ses chausses feust longue de troys piedz et quarrée, non ronde, ce que feust faict.* . . . Et disoit souvent que le monde n'avoit encores congneu l'émolument et utilité qui est de porter grande braguette; mais le temps leur enseigneroit quelque jour, comme

toutes choses ont esté inventées en temps. (*Pantagruel*, 15, 280/186; emphasis added)

And he had him dressed gallantly in the manner of the time it was then, *except that Panurge wanted the codpiece on his breeches to be three feet long and square, not round, which was done.* . . . And he often said that people had not yet recognized the advantage and utility there is in wearing a big codpiece; but time would teach them some day, even as in time all things have been invented.

Codpieces had undergone a radical transformation from the simple "round" (note Rabelais's text) to square, box-like shapes in a fashion change that roughly coincides with the outbreak and dissemination of syphilis in the years between the end of the fifteenth century and the first half of the sixteenth century. And what is more, it was a change that began with the soldiers and hired soldiers and even *gondolieri* in Italy and spread to the nobility—one of the rare instances, as Grace Q. Vicary notes, in which a radical change in fashion began with a lower class and was adopted by the highest rank—nobility: "The soft, triangular flap codpiece of the 15th century developed into a protruding, contorted, decorated enlarged, padded penis sheath that often matched the decorative forms displayed by the fashionably dressed men . . . of that time."[14] Vicary goes on to say that the earlier codpiece—worn in the fifteenth century—had a triangular, rounded flap "attached to the hose with laces and made of the same material as the hose, presumably washable. Next came stiffened, padded, protruding codpieces worn as additions matching either the hose or other clothing" (Vicary, 8). This last was worn in the sixteenth century and often curved backwards. Vicary provides portraits of the major kings of this time illustrating the padded, curved codpieces: Charles V, by Titian (1532); Henry VIII, presumably by Holbein (1537); and François I, by Clouet (1540). According to Vicary, the layers of woven cloth, made stiff with stays and padding, "formed a roomy box [so that] the genitals could rest inside, well protected from friction, bumps or knocks from the various daggers, purses, tools, whisks, pomanders, or swords which Renaissance men hung from their belts" (Vicary, 8).

Vicary suggests that the new codpiece contained both enough room for bandages and for the ointments that Rabelais's narrator mentions above. It concealed the male organ so that sores were not visible—providing a kind of a "camouflage from persecution" as well as a protection for other people in the crowded stores and streets so that they would not come into contact with the infected area (Vicary, 14). So, when Panurge specifies "la braguette de ses chausses feust longue de troys piedz et *quarrée,* non ronde [emphasis added]," he distinguishes the old style of codpiece from the new and asserts its practicality, which people would eventually come to understand (280/186). While adopting his prince's livery shows his fealty to Pantagruel, Panurge still asserts his right to follow fashion, particularly if in time one learns the usefulness of the new invention.

Panurge is never far from the pox, as is seen in chapter 16 of *Pantagruel,* in which he concocts a tart "Borbonnoise" made of excrement and pus from syphilis-infected pustules ("sanie de bosses chancreuses") to serve to passersby on a street (La rue de Fouarre) known to be frequented by master of arts students at the Sorbonne (*Pantagruel,* 16, 281, see also note 2, *Pantagruel,* 10, 256). The unsuspecting Parisians who feast on the tarts die of plague, leprosy, gout, and the greatest number from the pox.

We next see Panurge decked out in his new livery and codpiece at the debate with maistre Thaumaste (*Pantagruel,* ch. 18). Although Vicary could have looked elsewhere in Rabelais to support her ideas on the evolution of the codpiece, she limits her treatment of Rabelais to this one episode—but does a great service in resolving the issue of why Panurge should have an orange in his codpiece:

> Or notez que Panurge avoit mis au bout de sa longue braguette un beau floc de soye rouge, blanche, verte et bleue, et dedans avoit mis une belle pomme d'orange. (*Pantagruel,* ch. 18, 294/197)
>
> Now note that Panurge had put on the end of his long codpiece a lovely lock of silk, red, white, green, and blue, and inside it had put a fine orange.

Vicary disagrees with the English translation—a literal orange—and posits that the author was referring to a *pomme d'ambre,* pomander: "The original *pomme d'ambre* may have actually been carved from a ball of the harder resin, amber, which significantly, is dark-yellow in color. Second, Rabelais did not say *une belle orange* but *une belle pomme d'orange* (a beautiful head of an orange)." Her conclusion is that Rabelais was referring to the male sex organ as a head, colored orange—a reference to the mercury mixed with animal grease, a common treatment for syphilis. Remember the mercury mixed with vinegar and herbs mentioned by Paré, referenced above. "Thus, mercury salts combined with unrefined yellowish animal grease and used to treat syphilis would undoubtedly have turned the skin of the penis, orange, and any bandages used to dress the penis, orange" (Vicary, 17).

Vicary does not proceed to the next pertinent passage, in which Panurge takes the "pomme d'orange" and throws it seven times with his right hand, catching it on the eighth time, all the while extending his codpiece and shaking it with his left hand. This would suggest that the "pomme d'orange" is indeed a pomander—used for its fragrance based on aromatic herbs and spice in counterbalancing unpleasant smells, smells that could emanate from infection within the codpiece. Elizabeth Rodini advises us that it was thought that the strong scents from the pomander "had protective medicinal values: they would have warded off plague and disease, and sanitized the air."[15]

In any case, it seems that either Panurge was infected with the disease or was doing his best to ward off the disease. His advances toward the "haulte dame de Paris" would suggest the former rather than the latter. His victory over maistre Thaumaste raises his reputation among the Parisians such that he adds additional decoration to his codpiece:

> Panurge commença estre en réputation en la ville de Paris par ceste disputation que il obtint contre l'Angloys, et faisoit dès lors bien valoir sa braguette, et le feist au dessus esmoucheter de broderie à la romanicque. (*Pantagruel*, 21, 300/203)

> Panurge began to get a reputation around the town of Paris for this disputation he maintained against the Englishman, and from then on put his codpiece to good use, and had it decorated with Roman style embroidery.

We tend to imagine that intellectual capacity rather than virility leads to victory in disputation, but in Panurge's case he is emboldened to go above his social rank to throw his affections upon a married woman of high social rank. While he had argued with signs with Thaumaste, he is less successful in verbally making his case with the "haulte dame de Paris," particularly because his rhetoric betrays both his more humble origins and his lusty desires. Addressing himself to the lady, he says:

> Or (dist-il), ce me seroit bien tout un d'avoir bras et jambes couppez, en condition que nous fissions, vous et moy, un ranson de chère lie, jouans des manequins à basses marches, car (monstrant sa longue braguette)

voicy Maistre Jean Jeudy qui vous sonneroit une antiquaille dont vous sentirez jusques à la moelle des os. (*Pantagruel,* 21, 300/203)

Well, now, he said, it would be all the same to me to have my arms and legs cut off, on condition that you and I should have a nice roll in the hay together, playing the stiff lowdown in-and-out game; for (showing his long codpiece) here is Master Johnny Jumpup [Maistre Jean Jeudy], who will sound you an antic dance that you'll feel to the marrow of your bones.

Panurge's speech reveals the lowly milieu in which he generally seeks to satisfy his desires.[16] Lust and not the talent to create a true partnership with a woman leads Panurge to the fruitless quest for a wife in the *Tiers Livre,* or *Third Book.* But it is Rabelais's narrator who first presents the model of marriage based on a true give-and-take in *Gargantua,* in which the woman is capable of both taking pleasure in sexual relations and regretting those activities when faced with the pain of childbirth.

It is indeed fitting that a narrative that will lead to the birth and playful childhood of the giant Gargantua should be dedicated to the "Beuvers tres illustres, et vous Vérolez très précieux (car à vous, et non à aultres, sont dédiez mes escriptz)" (*Gargantua,* prologue, 38/3) [Most illustrious topers, and you, most precious poxies—for to you, not the others, my writings are dedicated]. The playful lovemaking, presumably focused on procreation, is the setting for the birth of Gargantua:

En son eage virile, [Grandgousier] espousa Gargamelle, fille du roy de Parpaillos, belle gouge et de bonne troigne, et faisoient eux deux souvent ensemble la beste à deux dos, joyeusement se frotans leur lard, tant qu' elle engroissa d'un beau filz et le porta jusques à la unziesme moys. (*Gargantua,* 3, 47/12)

In his prime, he married Gargamelle, daughter of the king of the Parpaillons, a good looking wench, and these two together often played the two-backed beat, so that she became pregnant with a handsome son and carried him until the eleventh month.

The subject of livery returns when it is time to dress the young Gargantua. Here again, the narrator mentions a change in sartorial style that would accommodate the more elaborate codpiece: "Pour son pourpoinct furent levées huyt cens treize aulnes de satin blanc, et pour les agueillettes quinze cens neuf peaulx et demye de chiens. *Lors commença le monde attacher les chausses au pourpoinct, et non le pourpoinct aux chausses"* (*Gargantua*, 60/22, emphasis added) [For his doublet were taken up eight hundred and thirteen ells of white satin, and for the points fifteen hundred and nine and a half dogskins. *Then people began to attach the hose to the doublet, and not the doublet to the hose*]. Gargantua, like Panurge, wears the more elaborate codpiece and doublet of the sixteenth century—where the protruding codpiece and hose underneath are attached to the doublet so that the codpiece can be removed for urination. Vicary remarks on this change: "Study of paintings and drawings indicate there was a major change in form of the padded, protruding codpiece. The first shape, found in Italian-Spanish portraits, was made of two oval pieces joined at center front which became an elongated padded flap attached to the long hose (1495, 1500, 1532 . . .)" (Vicary 9). Rabelais was clearly aware of changes in fashion brought about by the need to create larger, more elaborate codpieces, and he chose to comment on these changes repeatedly in his works. Rabelais's narrator continues to advance the novelty of the protruding codpiece:

> Pour la braguette feurent levées seize aulnes un quartier d'icelluy mesmes drap. Et fut la forme d'icelle comme d'un arc-boutant, bien estachée joyeusement à deux belles boucles d'or, que prenoient deux crochetz d'esmail, en un chascun desquelz estoyt enchassée un grosse esmeraude de la grosseur d'une pomme d'orange. (*Gargantua*, 8, 60/22–23; emphasis added)

> For the codpiece were taken up sixteen and a quarter ells of this same cloth. And the form of it was like a flying buttress, most merrily fastened with two beautiful gold buckles, caught up by two enamel hooks, in each of which was set a big emerald the size of an orange.

Rabelais appears to refer to codpieces "shaped into an upward and backward curved tube (similar to the mechanical French Curve)," a style popular in Germany, France, and England (Vicary, 9). Titian's portrait of Charles V, Holbein's portrait of Henry VIII, and Clouet's portrait of François I all exhibit the codpiece with the backward curve. While there is some evidence that all three monarchs, Charles V, Henry VIII, and François I, suffered from syphilis, Gargantua seems to have escaped the disease, but fashion had already dictated the style for codpieces to be worn by those who could afford the expense.[17] Such is the narrator's interest in the precise details of the codpiece, including the opening of the codpiece in blue damask, gold embroidery, diamonds, rubies, turquoises, and emeralds, that it suggests a cornucopia—"une corne d'abondance." This symbol of fecundity amidst such abundant details on the codpiece leads the narrator to promise to write another book, *De la dignité des braguettes,* a book he claims in the prologue to *Gargantua* (38/3) to already have written (Gargantua, 8, 61/23). Where livery is concerned, either for Panurge or Gargantua, the codpiece takes center stage.

Similarly, the absence of a codpiece becomes a preoccupation in the *Tiers Livre,* when Panurge gives up his codpiece to wear a monk-like robe at the very time he sets out on his marriage quest. Panurge maintains that the codpiece is primarily a mark of military dress—to protect the soldier in battle. This point of view coincides with the idea that the new fashion in codpieces had originated with the soldiers: "By 1500, when Italian soldiers were depicted in oval padded codpieces that were not yet worn by noblemen, and 1535 when the larger, backward-curved, padded codpieces appear in portraits of noblemen, extreme padded, protruding codpieces were depicted in drawings of Germanic mercenary soldiers (1525)" (Vicary, 10). Pantagruel takes exception to Panurge's assertion that the codpiece is the most essential piece of military wear: "Voulez-vous (dist Pantagruel) maintenir que la braguette est pièce première de harnois militaire? C'est doctrine moult paradoxe et nouvelle" (*Gargantua,* 8, 397) ["Do you mean," said Pantagruel, "to maintain that the codpiece is the first piece of military harness? That's a very paradoxical and novel doctrine"]. Pantagruel goes on to say that he thought spurs were more essential.

Panurge continues to advance his thesis on the necessity of the codpiece in protecting human sperm and thus the propagation of the human species, much as nature has provided protection for the reproductive organs of plants and animals. Returning to his thesis concerning the primacy of the codpiece in military wear, he cites verses from the *Chiabrena des pucelles* (1534) as the wife bids her husband not to forget to wear his codpiece to battle:

Celle qui veid son mary tout armé,
Fors la braguette, aller à l'escarmouche,
Luy dist: "Amy, de paour qu'on ne vous touche,
Armez cela, qui est le plus aymé." (*Le Tiers Livre,* 8, 399/281)

Seeing her husband armed from tip to toe,
Save for the codpiece, heading for the fray,
One woman said: "To keep you safe today,
My love, protect the part I cherish so."

For Pantagruel, it is Panurge's failure to follow "commun usaige," well-established custom, that displeases him: "Seulement me desplaist la nouveaulté et mespris du commun usaige" (*Le Tiers Livre*, 7, 395/278) [Only I don't like novelty and disdain for common usage]. Pantagruel views his friend's behavior as an aberration, an unexpected and disquieting change in behavior. For someone so fixed on maintaining his virility, Panurge abandons his "belle et magnificque braguette" for a dress or a monk's robe—both of which suggest a lack of sexual staying power. Pantagruel has become accustomed to Panurge's ornate codpiece, "en laquelle il souloit comme en l'ancre sacré constituer son dernier refuge contre tous naufraiges d'adversité" (394/277) [in which, as a holy anchor, he was wont to constitute his last refuge against all shipwrecks of adversity]. Its absence marks what will be the exchange of predictable behavior for a period of disturbing disequilibrium of long duration as Panurge weighs marriage and fatherhood against his fear of being cuckolded. The codpiece is a talisman of the friendship that is based on generosity, goodwill, and affection. In removing it along with the livery that was given him by Pantagruel and that was a measure of Panurge's fealty to his prince, he rejects this act of *caritas*—a gesture that Pantagruel finds disconcerting.

Elsewhere in *Gargantua*, as if to illustrate the ubiquity of the outbreak of syphilis in the general population, Rabelais's narrator recounts Gargantua's ingestion of the pilgrim, staff and all, with a leaf of salad. The pilgrim, in an attempt to test the unfamiliar geography of Gargantua's mouth, taps a nerve under one of the giant's teeth—causing great pain. Gargantua explores the painful area with a toothpick, with which he punctures a syphilitic chancre ("une bosse chancreuse"; *Gargantua*, ch. 38, 156/89) under the pilgrim's codpiece. The episode proves providential for the pilgrim, since he had been suffering from the pain of the tumor since "they had passed Ancenis" ("depuis le temps quíz eurent passé Ancenys"; 156/89).

Moving on to Panurge's dilemma in the *Tiers Livre*—his indecision as to whether he will marry—it can be seen that the fear of being cuckolded is linked to catching the pox. As he says, he has nothing against cuckolds but doesn't want to be one: "J'ayme bien les coquz, et me semble gens de bien . . . mais pour mourir je ne le vouldroys estre" (*Le Tiers*

Livre, 9, 400/282) [I like cuckolds perfectly well, and they seem like fine people to me . . . but for the life of me I wouldn't want to be one]. At this point in the debate over whether to marry or not, Panurge suggests that he marry an honest woman—not one who might beat him or worse, give him the pox: "N'est-ce le mieux que je me associe quelque honneste et preude femme, qu'ainsi changer de jour en jour avecques continuel dangier de quelque coup de baston, ou de la vérolle pour le pire? (401/283) [Isn't it better for me to take on with some good worthy woman, rather than change from day to day with continual danger of a beating or at the worst the pox?]. Yet he is the first to admit that he hasn't pursued or desired virtuous women—and even these might beat him or cuckold him, "car femme de bien oncques ne me feut rien" (401/283) [for no decent women ever meant anything to me]. Panurge is stuck in his habits of pursuing women who are most likely to deceive him and hence, in the present climate, give him the pox.

It is the *Quart Livre* that is the most focused on medicine: the demeanor of the doctor, the doctor's ability to tend to his own health, and the image of Christ, as reflected in Saint Luke, chapter 4:23, as the Christus medicus.[18] The tone is set from the letter to Odet de Coligny, a letter that appears in the edition of 1552, but not in the first partial edition of 1548, in which Rabelais asked for his protection against the "calumniateurs" who attacked his works. In the letter, he describes the role of the physician as one member in a farce, where the sickness and the patient are the other two players (letter to Monseigneur Odet, cardinal de Chastillon, *Le Quart Livre,* 562). He cites Johannes Alexandrinus's commentary on Hippocrates on the importance of the physician's dressing so as not to offend or disturb the patient: "mais pour le gré du malade duquel je visite, auquel seul je veulx enièrement complaire, en rien ne l'offenser ne fascher" (563/422) [but for the taste of the patient I am visiting, whom alone I want to please entirely, not offend or vex him in any way]. Hippocrates, Rabelais states, extolled the virtue of bringing a cheerful face to the bedside of the sick person rather than a sad or severe mien. The expression of the physician will either upset or reassure the patient, and Rabelais credits Plato and Averrois with this opinion. The words of the physician to the patient must have a single goal: "c'est le resjouir sans offense de Dieu et ne le contrister en façon quelconques" (564/422) [that is to gladden him without offense to God and not to sadden him in any way whatever].[19]

This letter prepares the way for Rabelais's view of the physician's role in the midst of a medical crisis—a philosophy that he describes in the 1552 prologue to the *Quart Livre, Pantagruélisme:* "Vous entendez que c'est certaine gayeté d'esprit conficte en mespris des choses fortuites" ("Prologue de l'Autheur," 368/425) [You understand that that's a certain gayety of spirit confected in disdain for fortuitous things]. The prologue opens with an address not to the "Beuveurs très illustres & Goutteux très précieux" of the prologue of the 1548 short edition of the *Quart Livre, Gargantua* and the *Tiers Livre,* but to the "Gens de bien, Dieu vous saulve et guard!" (568/425) [Good people, God save and guard you!]. The narrator puts off reference to chancres and syphilitics until much farther along in the prologue in order to inquire about the health of his readers. In turn, he maintains that he, thanks to his philosophy of *Pantagruélisme,* is "sain et dégourt, prest à boire" (568/425) [healthy, and sprightly, ready to drink].

The narrator's own state of health—and here most readers would make the extra-textual connection between the narrator and Rabelais as physician—leads him into a citation that has both biblical and medical connections. He cites Saint Luke 4:23: "Médecin, o guériz toy-mesmes" (568/425) [Physician, heal thyself]. Not content to leave the authority to just the Bible, he cites the concordance between Saint Luke and other authorities: Euripides cited by Galen, Erasmus, and Tiraqueau: "Médecin est des aultres en effect; / Toutesfois est d'ulcères tout infect" (569/426) [Although he treats others to good effect, / His running sores attest his self-neglect]. For the sixteenth-century reader, the running sores of course evoke the pox. Rabelais cites the renowned physician of the second century BCE, Asclepiades, to reinforce the previous authorities: "que médecin réputé ne feust, si malade avoit esté depuys le temps qu'il commença practiquer l'art jusques sa dernière vieillesse" (569/426) [that he should be reputed no doctor if he had ever been sick from the time he began to practice his craft until his final old age].

It is at this moment, having grounded his point of view in classical authorities, that he evokes the Augustinian concept of the Christus medicus in healing the faithful. Marjorie O'Rourke Boyle reminds us that this was also a treasured image of Erasmus, who when writing to Henry VIII to discourage him from an alliance with Charles V against France, advises Henry to favor the health of the body politic in seeking peace rather than war. Continuing to follow Erasmus's thought, she remarks: "The Lord Jesus was a physician who by speaking expelled atrocious and inveterate diseases, even resurrecting the dead."[20] Embedded in this concept is the idea that Christ's power surpasses all human craft and knowledge:

Si, par quelque désastre, s'est Santé de vos seigneuries émancipée, quelque part, dessus, dessoubz, davant, darière, à dextre, à senestre, dedans, dehors, loing ou près vos territoires qu'elle soit, la puissiez-vous incontinent avecques l'ayde du benoist Servateur rencontrer! (569/426)

If by some disaster Health has emancipated herself from your lordships, above, beneath, to the right, to the left, within, without, far from your territories or near them, wherever she may be, may you, with the help of the blessed Savior, promptly come upon her!

There follows a praise of health—and ample praise of André Tiraqueau and Henry II—for the role health plays in life: "Sans santé n'est la vie vivable" ("Without health life is not life, life is not livable") he says, quoting Aristophanes (969).

The subject of health and moderate wishes eventually leads, after several intervening tales, to the health of the "goutteux" and to the narrator's affection for them and hope that their health will be restored:

C'est goutteux, sus quoy je fonde mon espérance, et croy fermement que, s'il plaist au bon Dieu, vous obtiendrez santé, veu que rien plus que santé pour le présent me demandez. Attendez encores un peu, avecques demie once de patience. (581/435)

That, gouties is what I base my hope on, and I firmly believe that, if the good God please, you will obtain health. Wait a little longer, with half an ounce of patience.

The appearance of the gouty ones does not appear without thematic precedent, especially in the double interpretation of "coingnée," the hatchet lost by the woodcutter. Priapus attests that it has more than one meaning:

Je notay que ceste diction, coingnée, est équivoque à plusieurs choses. Elle signifie un certain instrument par le service duquel est fendu et couppé boys. Signifie aussi . . . la femelle bien à poinct et souvent gimbretiltolletée, et veidz que tout bon compaignon appelloit sa guarse fille de joye: ma coingnée. Car, avecques cestuy ferrement (cela disoit exhibant son coingnouoir dodrental) ilz leur coingnent. (576/431)

I noted that the term *coingnée* [modern *cognée*] is ambiguous, meaning several things. It means . . . the female fully ripe and frequently copiocopulated [*gimbretiletolletée*]; and I saw what each good fellow called his merry girlfriend *ma coingnée*. For with this naked steel (this he said exhibiting his half-cubit knocker) they knock [them] up.

This is indeed the popular arena in which the pox is spread. Yet, with the narrator/physician's hope that the gouty ones recover their health, the healing process can begin with the reading of the tales of the *Quart Livre de Pantagruel*: "Or, en bonne santé toussez un bon coup, beuvez en trois, secouez dehaiat vos aureilles, et vous oyrez dire merveilles du noble et bon Pantagruel" (582/435) [Now, in good health cough one good cough, drink three drinks, give your ears a cheery shake, and you shall hear wonders about the good and noble Pantagruel]. As in the tale of Panurge's dispute with maistre Thaumaste mentioned earlier (Pantagruel 19/20), where Panurge advances his luck with his codpiece on the basis of his victory in the verbal and mental disputation, Priapus continually substitutes *mentula* for "memory": "Et me soubvient (car j'ay mentule, voyre diz-je mémoire)" [And I remember (for I have a mentula, or rather I mean memory]; "ô belle mentule, voire, diz-je mémoire!" [O lovely mentula, or rather memory!] (576–77/431). In Rabelais's world, as Bakhtin has stated, mind and sex organ are often interchangeable. Reproduction is at the base of the survival of the species. As Panurge expounds in *Le Tiers Livre*, chapter 8: "La teste perdue ne perist que la personne: les couilles perdues périroit toute humaine nature" (399/281) [The head lost, perishes only the person, the balls lost, would perish all human nature]. It is understandable that it should be Priapus who reminds us of the essential nature of fertility in the perpetuation of the human species. Neither Rabelais nor the other physicians of the time were blind to the role that syphilis played in threatening fertility and the power of those infected to reproduce. The struggles of the royal families in Europe to produce healthy heirs was a reminder of the threat disease brought to successful reproduction. In her article "Bronzino's London Allegory and the Art of Syphilis," Margaret Healy comments that Erasmus was so concerned about the spread of syphilis and the decrease in fertility that he wrote four dialogues devoted to the topic. He "was calling—through the voices of his protagonists—for active measures to control it."[21]

It was not merely that a substantial portion of the population was not propagating the species because of vows of celibacy but also that noncelibate individuals who were engaged in wanton sexual practices put the entire population at risk. In a letter to the chancellor of Poland written in 1525, Erasmus states, as cited by Healy: "What sickness has ever traversed every part of Europe, Africa, and Asia with equal speed? What clings more tenaciously? What repels more vigorously the art and care of physicians? What passes more easily by contagion to another? What brings more cruel tortures?"[22] Gargantua's plea near the end of *Le Tiers Livre* that his son Pantagruel marry seems to reflect, in contrast to Panurge's combination of unbridled lust and blind fear and indecision at the prospect of marriage, his concern for providing a healthy succession to the kingdom: "Je loue Dieu, filz très cher, qui vous conserve en désirs vertueux, et me plaist très bien que par vous soit le voyage perfaict. Mais je vouldroys que pareillement vous vint en vouloir et désir vous marier" (*Le Tiers Livre*, 48, 537/398) [I praise God, my very dear son, for keeping you in virtuous desires, and I'm very pleased to have you complete this journey. But I'd like to see you too come to the will and desire to marry]. God has kept his son on the path of virtue. He makes it clear, as Pantagruel has done before him, that Panurge's path is quite different. Panurge suffers from a problem of will: "Panurge s'est assez efforcé rompre les difficultez qui luy pouvoient estre un empeschement." (538/398) [Panurge has striven enough to break down the difficulties that could have been an obstacle to him]. As I have said elsewhere, Panurge lacks the insight based on faith to put his fate in God's hands, and to align his will with God's will so that he is secure in his choice.[23] Gargantua praises Pantagruel for letting divine will guide him. The son cannot imagine another path for him:

> Pere très débonnaire (respondit Pantagruel), encores n'y avoys-je pensé: de tout ce négoce, je m'en deportoys sus vostre bonne volonté et paternel commendement. Plustost prie Dieu estre à vos piedz roydde mort en vostre desplaisir que, sans vostre plaisir, estre veu vif marié. (*Le Tiers Livre*, 48, 538/398)

> "My very kind father," replied Pantagruel. "I hadn't yet given it a thought. I was referring all that business to your goodwill and paternal command. I pray to God rather to be seen stone dead for having displeased you than without your pleasure to be seen alive and married."

The reader is pulled into the controversy of priests and monks interfering with the parents' right to choose suitable spouses for their children. Evangelical reform, opposing views of the family, and the new threat of an epidemic that puts reproduction and the rights of family succession at risk intersect as themes in the contrast between Pantagruel and Panurge in Rabelais's work.

One of the early episodes of the *Quart Livre* pits the sheep merchant Dindenault against Panurge. Not tricked by Panurge's disguise with the codpiece ("sans braguette") and with his glasses on his bonnet ("avecques ses lunettes attachées au bonnet"), the merchant knows a cuckold when he sees one: "Voyez-là une belle médaille de Coqu" (*Le Quart Livre*, ch. 5, 595/447) [That's a nice picture of a cuckold]. Panurge's reply reinforces the lust that drives his thoughts about women; he challenges the merchant to imagine that he found Panurge seducing his wife. The portrait of Panurge "sacksackshakeshookbingbangasspassed" the respectable wife of the merchant is an act of pure bravado on Panurge's part:

> Je te demande (dist Panurge) si, par consentement et convenance de tous les éléments, j'avoys sacsacbezevesinemassé ta tant belle, tant advenente, tant honeste, tant preude femme, de mode que le roydde dieu des jardins Priapus, lequel icy habite en liberté, subjection forcluse de braguettes attachées, luy feust on corps demeuré, en tel désastre que jamais n'en sortiroit, éternellement y resteroit, sinon que tu le tirasses avecques les dens, que feroys-tu? (596/448)

> "I ask you this," said Panurge: "if by the consent and agreement of all the elements, I had sacksackshakeshookbinbbangasspassed your ever so beautiful, ever so decent, ever so modest wife, to such effect that that stiff god of the gardens Priapus (who dwells here at liberty, subjection to codpieces being excluded) had remained stuck in her body so disastrously that it would never come out unless you pulled it out with your teeth, what would you do?"

Panurge's provocation leads to Dindenault's efforts to pull out his sword, but in an act worthy of farce, it sticks in the scabbard. Nonetheless, Panurge lacks the courage to take him on and runs for cover next to Pantagruel. Frère Jan, ironically the most virile and soldier-like of the company, would have done the merchant in. Panurge's words do not match his actions on this journey, as evidenced by his taking cover during a major storm that besets the crew in chapter 18: Panurge "restoit acropy sus le tillac, tout affligé, tout meshaigné et à demy mort; invocqua tous les benoistz sainctz et sainctes à son ayde" (*Le Quart Livre*, ch. 18, 633/478) [remained squarring on deck, all upset, all beat, and half dead, invoked all the blessed saints, men and women to his aid].

Panurge's earlier adventures with women of unsavory character, and his thoughts, which reinforce either his past actions or his lusty desires, make him a figure at risk for contracting syphilis. Whether his abandonment of the codpiece signals a sincere desire to find a suitable wife or a loss of sexual prowess as a result of past actions, his search for the woman of "semblable température" in order to produce offspring "dignes de quelque monarchie transpontine" is unlikely to bear fruit (*Le Tiers Livre*, ch. 31, 486/354). His friends, Pantagruel, Gargantua, Frère Jan, and Epistemon, see only too clearly their friend's unsuitability for the institution of marriage. Rabelais, like Erasmus, looks to the guidance that Pantagruel receives from his father and from his young giant's spiritual upbringing to conserve the nobility and the monarchy from the ravages of the pox. Evangelical humanism places the family in a central position for the social and spiritual education of the child. For Rabelais, as for Erasmus, the church plays a role in this regard, but the parents have a responsibility not to be shirked in guiding the social and spiritual path of the offspring.[24]

The outbreak of syphilis in Europe at the end of the fifteenth century affected every aspect of life and demanded changes in hygiene, medical treatment, clothing, the circulation of people, and the interactions of the social classes. Rabelais's work gives periodic glimpses of the ways in which Europeans adapted to the presence and spread of this disease. As a physician, Rabelais recorded the impact, but as a storyteller, he realized the potential that the disease could serve as a metaphor for approaching life and the treatment of disease. The pox leveled the social hierarchy in attacking kings and peasants, learned and illiterate individuals alike. In doing so, the disease took center stage in prompting calls for innovative responses in every corner of society: on the battlefield, among pilgrims, among students and learned clerks and professors, and among courtiers, kings, and princes. The following chapter reveals how Erasmus took up some of the same themes treated by Rabelais and focused on the importance of health within the family unit to ensure both the physical and spiritual well-being of future generations in Europe.

2

Erasmus, *The Colloquies*, and Syphilis

SEVERAL FACTORS in Erasmus's life make his writing a lens through which to observe the pandemic of syphilis in the early part of the sixteenth century: he travelled widely in Europe to France, Switzerland, Italy, Germany, and the Low Countries; was in correspondence with physicians; and wrote about the spread of the disease he witnessed across the countries he visited. Indeed, the *Colloquies* return on numerous occasions to the rapid spread of the disease, the danger faced both by those stricken with the disease and those who live in proximity to diseased patient, and, finally, possible ways to stop the spread of the disease. As a relatively young man, Erasmus saw the introduction of the disease in Europe and watched as it reached a period of particular virulence before his death in 1536. Franz Bierlaire comments on the filiation between Erasmus's *Colloquies* and the events of his time: "Everything that happens in his daily life goes into the mix."[1]

While the previous chapter of this book analyzed in detail the treatment that Rabelais gave the disease—both literally and as a metaphor—the present chapter will explore how Erasmus weaves the topic of syphilis into the much broader fabric of the *Colloquies*. In the process of the analysis, I will relate the topic of syphilis to several other subjects he treats: war and peace, territorial expansion along with the treatment of conquered peoples, religious controversy, and the relationship of husbands and wives as well as their roles in the upbringing of their children.

Barbara Cornell focuses her study of the *Colloquies* on those dialogues that present

> Erasmus grappling with two important issues and relating them to a mutable text of identity in the early modern civil subject: the dangerous problems of women's power and the instability of adolescence as the treacherous, limited period when the boy appropriates his sexual identity as the prerequisite to entering the civic realm.[2]

The topics of courtship and marriage, along with those colloquies that make up what she terms the "marriage group," are central to the problems posed by the spread of syphilis, as shall be seen in Erasmus's treatment of syphilis in "A Marriage in Name Only." So, too, the risks that mothers ran in giving up their newborn infants to wet nurses, a topic of "The New Mother," were known to Erasmus as well as to competent physicians and surgeons of the period in which syphilis began spreading across Europe.[3] His focus on the role of knights and soldiers in spreading syphilis as they travelled from one site of conflict to another leads him to condemn parents who would sacrifice the well-being of their daughters for the sake of acquiring aristocratic titles. Syphilis is a scourge that threatens the family structure and the generation of healthy children, and the *Colloquies* bear witness to sound practices in preparing young people to assume the role of constructive participants in society. The themes that Rabelais treats in narrative form, Erasmus examines through the still familiar but more philosophical form of dialogue; courtship, marriage, childbearing, childrearing, adolescence, and education are topics. Both authors were observers of the rapid spread of the pox in the first part of the sixteenth century, and both explore the literal and figurative impact of the disease on European society.

Erasmus's choice of the colloquy as a form to treat matters that are both fundamental to civil structure and yet intimate—high in importance but familiar in content—means that he can include within its format topics relating to the individual's most personal nature: intimate relations, sexually transmitted diseases, bad breath, whoring, hygiene or lack thereof. Scholars of Erasmus agree that the genius of his colloquies is to combine elements of the Ciceronian, Socratic, and Lucianic models to allow the satirical aspect of the Lucianic model to enliven yet not diminish the persuasive elements inherent to the Ciceronian and Socratic models.[4]

As Eva Kushner so ably demonstrates, the *Colloquies* come to life because each participant in the dialogue speaks some truth. Such a strategy prevents the conversations from being a dull, pedagogical exercise. The irony provides a kind of suspense leading only eventually to the key concept against which the persistent antagonist has been arguing: "Grâce à l'ironie, un certain 'suspense' y guide le cheminement de l'idée privilégiée à travers l'épaisseur de la résistance de l'antagoniste" (Kushner, 20). If the views of each interlocutor have no ring of truth, then the conversation loses its dynamism.

For the purposes of this study, it is important to note Kushner's observation that Erasmus views the dialogue, and in particular his *Colloquies,* as the recounting of a conversation leading to a solution, and she credits Rudolf Hirzel with this definition of the dialogue.[5] The discussion of specific colloquies to follow takes into account that Erasmus evokes the disease in order to work out some manner of slowing down its disastrous course through Europe. By approaching the disease and its perils from the diverse points of view of the interlocutors, Erasmus seeks to offer some credible solutions. As Kushner states, he respects the aesthetic necessity of reconciling what is useful with what gives pleasure (Kushner, 21).

Let us turn now to individual colloquies in which Erasmus turns to reference the new epidemic, the French or Spanish pox, *grosse vérole,* or *bubas,* among other names. Barbara Cornell notes that the various colloquies were composed "over decades" from 1496 to 1529—precisely the time that physicians in Europe noted the outbreak of syphilis following the return of Columbus's sailors to Europe and the crowds of soldiers and mercenaries in Italy at the time of France's invasion of Italy.[6] In his *Histoire de la syphilis: Son origine, son expansion,* Jeanselme notes that the witness whose testimony carries the most weight ("dont le témoignage a le plus de poids") was Gonzalo Fernández de Oviedo y Valdés because he followed the outbreak from the Court of Spain, where he was attached to Don Juan, son of the Spanish monarchs, and was in contact with the companions of Admiral Christopher Columbus and then served in the Spanish army in Naples when Charles VIII invaded Naples. He comments that this was the first time that the disease had been observed in Italy. From there he was sent to the New World, where he could observe that the Indians were not as severely affected by *las bubas* or pox as the European soldiers and mercenaries had been in Italy.[7]

In the order in which the various colloquies of Erasmus appear, "The Soldier and the Carthusian" ("Militis et Cartusiani") is the first in which syphilis is mentioned. Erasmus is consistent with the medical and historical writings of the time in attributing the spread of the pox to the itinerant lives of the soldiers. In her analysis of this particular dialogue, Eva Kushner credits Erasmus with not immediately giving moral authority to the Chartreux monk and so respecting at the beginning of the dialogue the Ciceronian model where both voices stand on equal ground.[8] At the outset and until just before the conclusion of the conversation, the Carthusian and the soldier argue with equal vehemence about the superiority of their way of life. The Chartreux notes that he has a more pleasant existence because he serves a good prior, while the soldier is slave to the whims of a "barbarous officer" (CWE, 39: 333). The soldier finds fault with the confined life of the Carthusian—an existence that restricts both where he can go and what he can do. He pities the Carthusian for having to shave his head, but the latter notes that a shaved head is more hygienic and more convenient (CWE, 39: 330).

Through this verbal competition, the moral authority of the Carthusian comes to light only toward the end of the colloquy, where he points out the radically changed physical appearance of his friend, the soldier. The scars caused by a splinter of a crossbow that hit him in the forehead only add to the disfiguration caused by the ravages of the pox. "Well, I notice some sort of ornaments on your chin, too," observes the Carthusian (CWE, 39: 334). Amidst the soldier's attempts to discount the red marks, the Carthusian says that he suspects that the soldier has had the pox. The soldier admits that it is the third time he has had the disease and this last time nearly lost his life (CWE, 39: 334). His friend notes his stooping stature—the result of the joint problems known to be caused by the pox—an observation confirmed by the soldier: "The disease contracted the joints" (CWE, 39: 334).

Having worn his interlocutor down, the Carthusian brings the conversation back to his friend's metamorphosis from a horseman to "a creeping creature instead of a centaur" (CWE, 39: 335). Erasmus underscores the fall from human to subhuman species by the Latin phrase "animal semi-reptile" (OO, I-3: 318). The Carthusian speculates that the pox has taken on a fashionable aura because it is so widespread among the nobility. It is here that the Carthusian exerts his moral authority and where we observe Erasmus's opposition to war and the errant life of the soldier precisely because it places the innocent family of the infected soldier at great risk. In response to the soldier's statement that his illness and wounds are the "chances of war," the Carthusian responds: "And what prizes do you bring home to your wife and children? Now you will infect with this disease those what ought to be most precious to you, and you yourself will go through life a rotten corpse" (CWE, 39: 335). The monk turns from the physical symptoms of syphilis to the moral attack on the soldier's soul caused by his wandering, whoring, and other unhealthy activities in the urban centers of Europe. He brings back a putrid, scabied soul to his wife and children. The Latin, rather than Craig Thompson's translation, captures the metaphor for the scabied or ulcered soul: "Iam animam vero qualem reportas, quanta scabie putrem, quot vulneribus sauciam?" (OO, I–3: 319) [But what kind of soul will you bring back? Rotten with how many diseases? Torn by how many wounds? (CWE, 39: 335)]. Begging his friend to stop chiding him, the soldier requests food, a request granted through the charity of the priory.

The sanctity of the family and the welfare of the children are at the core of Erasmus's colloquy. His words suggest that the soldier's pox is not only transmittable to the wife through sexual relations but to the children, unborn or through nursing. I will later reflect on the dangers of sending out infants to be nursed by unhealthy wet nurses by exploring the dialogue "The New Mother." Civil and religious strife and the ambition of monarchs give rise to the need for mercenary soldiers, and this message comes through in the colloquy above. The immediate implied solution is to put an end to war so that soldiers will not wander, and in so doing, infect their families with this new disease. As the Carthusian suggests, war reduces soldiers to animals (semi-reptiles) by transforming both body and soul to rot. The solution here is implicit rather than explicit. Franz Bierlaire comments on the increasing force with which Erasmus had been sounding the alarm in his works since the resumption of hostilities between Charles V and Francis I.[9] In other colloquies, the message will be more direct and turns around the social structures.

If war leads to itinerant soldiers, the need for inns becomes all the more present. In the dialogue "Inns" ("Diversoria"), suggestions are made to indicate that inns are indeed a breeding place for the pox because of the familiar exchanges among guests in cramped quarters. "Laughing, jolly, sporting girls everywhere" (CWE, 39: 370) [puellae ridentes, lasciviantes, lusitantes (OO, I–3: 334)] interact with the male guests at the inn. Erasmus uses the adjective "lascivantes" to describe the young women's sporting behavior rather than Thompson's less suggestive "jolly." The innkeeper's wives and daughters take liberties with their guests in talking with them "not as strangers" but "as with old familiar friends" (CWE 39: 370). The common air, with many people crowded in a single place, is conducive to contagion, and in particular, to passing on the pox. William, in talking with Bertulph, expounds on the dangers:

But nothing seems to be more dangerous than for so many persons to breathe the same warm air, especially when their bodies are relaxed and they've eaten together and stayed in the same place a good many hours. Quite apart from the belching of garlic, the breaking of wind, the stinking breaths, many persons suffer from hidden diseases, and every disease is contagious. Undoubtedly many have the Spanish or, as some call it, French pox, though it's common to all countries. (CWE, 39: 372)

The solution here seems to be to avoid such common places and at the very least, change the sheets with greater frequency:

> BERTULPH: Then everyone is shown to his nest. Actually a mere cubicle, since it contains only beds and nothing else you could use or steal.
> WILLIAM: Is it clean?
> BERTULPH: Like dinner: the linen washed perhaps six months before.
> (CWE, 39: 375)

The mobile citizenry breaks down the social structure, with both mixing of socioeconomic classes and confusion of social behavior: strangers being treated as intimates, wanton behavior taking place between young women and guests whom they had just met at the inn. This confusion is added to by the mix of ethnic customs: German, French, Italian, and English (a hybrid of French and German customs, comments William; CWE, 39: 375).

"The Young Man and the Harlot" ("Adolescentis et Scorti") sets in play a dialogue, somewhat like that of "The Soldier and the Carthusian," in which Lucretia the harlot and Sophronius the young man converse on the price that Lucretia has paid for abandoning her real family—"father, mother, brothers, sisters, paternal and maternal aunts"—for life in the brothel, a place that would bring shame on her family (CWE, 39: 383). She counters his logic by stating: "Oh, no, I have exchanged my loved ones, to my profit, for instead of a few I now have many—of whom you are one. I've always looked upon you as a brother" (CWE, 39: 384). Sophronius entreats her to pay heed to Christ's redemption and to save herself before the pox takes her: "And if you haven't yet caught the new contagion called the Spanish pox [scabiem Hispanicam] you can't long escape it" (CWE, 39: 384/OO, I-3: 341). He reasons that she has exchanged one form of servitude—to her family—for another: "You used to think obeying your mother burdensome, now you're at the beck and call of an utterly repulsive bawd" (CWE, 39: 384). Recall the Carthusian's similar reproach to the soldier, when the former mentioned that the soldier must obey "a barbarous officer" while the monk follows the lead of a "good" prior (CWE, 39: 333).

Sophronius explains that he followed the advice of his confessor in Rome, who advised him: "Son, if you truly repent and change your way of life, I don't care much about penance. But if you persist, lust itself will exact more than enough penance from you, even if the priest does not impose it. Look at me: blear-eyed, palsied, stooped" (CWE, 39: 385–86). The confessor assesses the damage done by the pox to the young man. The efficacy of the cure lies not in the pilgrimage to Rome but in the sincerity of the repentance and the depth of belief.

Impressed by the transformation of the young man from debauched to chastened and faithful, converted upon his visit to a confessor in Rome, Lucretia accepts his offer to support her while she chooses a more chaste path—either marriage or sacred vows or employment with "the family of some respectable housewife" (CWE, 39: 386). As in the outcome of "The Soldier and the Carthusian," it takes a well-meaning act of charity to convince Lucretia to mend her wanton ways. By pointing out that there was more than one way—prostitution—to provide for herself, Sophronius offers a palette of choices that provide an honest way to survive. Youthful desire to escape the yoke of the family has led Lucretia to make a bad choice, one that will shorten her life and corrupt her soul.[10] It takes but a modest and sincere act of charity to open her to more honest options.[11]

Earlier in this chapter, I noted that Erasmus reacted harshly to wars of expansion and to the rapid spread of the pox that the frequent movement of military troops and the growth of military camps have caused. He denounced the damage done by the absence of the fathers and sons from their families and the subsequent infection brought back to the families by the soldiers. Marriage and family lie at the heart of Christian society for Erasmus in terms of forming children to assume their rightful place in the civil structure. As noted in the discussion of "The Soldier and the Carthusian," the risks of disease and disability that come from war put the ones who are dearest to the soldier at greatest peril—in terms of both health and income (CWE, 39: 335). Erasmus begins the colloquy "The New Mother" with Eutrapelus congratulating Fabulla on the birth of her son, but he follows his congratulations by a long harangue on world conflict, covering the imprisonment of François I, the expansionism of Charles V, the hunger inflicted on the populations of Europe by the military strife, factionalism in religious orders, and controversy over the Eucharist (CWE, 39: 592).

World conflict between rulers and church figures is mirrored by conflict in the microcosm of the family—the role played by the mother in nursing her child or in giving her child to the wet nurse. Fabulla yields to the advice of friends "because they thought a person as young as I am should not be nursing" and so gives the baby to be suckled by a wet nurse (CWE, 39: 595). Eutrapelus argues in favor of nature: "But if nature gave you strength to conceive, undoubtedly it gave you strength to nurse, too" (CWE, 39: 595). He takes a line of logic that asks Fabulla if she would consent to have another called the mother of her child. She responds, "Not for the world!" Eutrapelus continues: "Then why are you willing to transfer more than half of the name of mother to some other woman?" (CWE, 9: 595). Eutrapelus points out that nature has all mothers care for their young—whether owls, lions, or vipers. To her reply that she is indeed her son's sole mother, her interlocutor replies: "No, Fabulla, nature herself contradicts you on that score" (CWE, 39: 595).[12]

It becomes clear that it is not only for reasons of nurturing but for reasons of health—wholesomeness—that Eutrapelus urges Fabulla to nurse her child herself rather than summon a wet nurse.

> Or isn't it a kind of exposure to hand over the tender infant, still red from its mother, drawing breath from its mother, crying for its mother's care—a sound said to move even wild beasts—to a woman who perhaps has neither good health or good morals and who, finally, may be much more concerned about a bit of money than about your whole baby? (CWE, 39: 595–96)

To Fabulla's response that "the woman chosen is of sound health," Eutrapelus lets her know that the doctors think otherwise. The most wholesome and natural thing is for the child to drink its mother's milk—what is familiar—related in blood and upbringing: "But assume that she's equal to you in this respect, or better, if you like. Do you suppose it makes no difference whether a delicate infant drinks in congenial and familiar nourishment and is cherished by the now familiar warmth or is forced to get used to somebody else's?" (CWE, 39: 596). The humanist plays on the contrast between "familiar" and "alien"/"strange" ("familiarem" as opposed to "alienis"; OO, I-3: 458).

Erasmus was more vehement than some in his belief that women should nurse their own children. He shared the opinion of surgeons who practiced in the late fifteenth and sixteenth centuries who recorded problems that came from using wet nurses whose health was in question. These surgeons wrote in the vernacular and "had contact with young children in the course of their work, unlike physicians who tended at this time to lack experience with infants and left their care to midwives and surgeons."[13] Nicholas Terpstra comments, "Among children, the greatest dangers were to nursing infants, who could pick up the infection as they suckled."[14] It was the surgeons who most often treated cases of syphilis, and so they would have witnessed the communication of syphilis to the babies suckled by wet nurses infected with the disease. It was also true that returning soldiers, knights, or well-off urban professionals could infect their wives with the disease, and so these mothers would in turn infect their babies, who would then infect an innocent wet nurse with the pox. Eutrapelus seeks to counsel Fabulla to follow nature's way in imparting her presumed healthy constitution to her newborn child—since any change from the accustomed presence of his mother may harm his well-being.

Eutrapelus suggests as well that the child absorbs the moral character as well as the wholesome body of the mother: "He needs that now familiar, recognized fluid which he has absorbed in her body and by which he grew strong. And for my part, I'm convinced that children's characters are injured by the nature of the milk just as in fruits or plants the moisture of the soil changes the quality which it nourishes" (CWE, 39: 605; emphasis added). The virtuous presence of the mother will shape the honest character of the child in its early years. Valerie Fildes notes: "The belief that babies ingested the mental and physical characteristics of the woman or animal who fed them was still very strong, and was one reason for avoiding animal milks, except in an emergency" (Fildes, 73). This is a belief that persists a half century later, and is mentioned in Montaigne's *Essais*, book 2, chapter 8, where he recounts seeing goats recognize the cry of the child they have suckled or the child refuse the milk of any but the goat who has suckled it.[15]

In her treatment of the colloquy of "The New Mother," Barbara Cornell comments on the established role of the mother in "her moulding duties, gently nurturing the child as is appropriate for the first years of life" (Cornell, 255). Erasmus's condemnation, through the persona of Eutrapelus, of the practice of sending well-bred children to the wet nurse on the basis of hygiene as well as on the basis of wholesome and honest upbringing leads one to think of his contemporary, François Rabelais, a physician himself. When Gargamelle gives birth to Gargantua, the narrator suggests that because of his large size and healthy thirst, 17,913 cows were ordered from fertile villages in proximity to the author's home in Chinon to provide him milk ("dix et sept mille neuf cens treze vaches de

Pautille et de Brehemond pour l'alaicter ordinairement").[16] Given what has been said above about the preference for the mother's nursing of the child and the reluctance to give animal milk to children lest they be deprived of the mother's nurturing, why does Rabelais suggest that Gargantua was not nursed by his mother? Rabelais hedges his bets, perhaps a nod to the learned Erasmus, giving an alternative story that would have Gargamelle nurse her own child:

> For it was impossible to find an adequate wet nurse in the whole countryside, considering the great quantity of milk required to feed him, although certain Scotist doctors have asserted that his mother nursed him and that she could draw from her breasts fourteen hundred and two casks and nine pipes of milk each time, which is not likely, and the proposition was declared mammalogically scandalous, offensive to pious ears, and smacking from afar of heresy.[17]

The reader is left with the possibility that the prince was nursed by his mother, but knows that because of his large size and appetite, it is highly unlikely that Gargamelle actually had the capacity attributed to her. We might imagine the author—along with the readers—delighting in the grotesque imagery of Gargamelle's enormous breasts and the prospect of the learned and censoring educators at the Sorbonne being themselves accused of heresy for inventing such a tall tale. After all, it was Noël Béda and his fellow theologians at the Sorbonne who condemned Erasmus's *Colloquies* on May 16, 1526, a prelude to their attacks on Rabelais's works in the next decade.[18]

Nevertheless, Erasmus is definite in his admonition against using a wet nurse. He, as well as his correspondent Rabelais, would have been only too aware of the dangers of transmission of the pox through breast milk. The outbreak of syphilis in Europe posed a threat to the foundational social structure represented by the family. For this reason, Eutrapelus urges Fabulla to safeguard the health and well-being of her child by nursing him herself and giving up the practice of the wet nurse. To her justification that giving the child to a wet nurse is "common practice" ("vulgo fit"; OO, I-3: 417), her interlocutor reasons, "You name the worst authority on good behavior, Fabulla; sinning is common, gambling is common, visiting brothels is common; cheating, boozing, folly are common" (CWE, 39: 595). The solution to keeping a healthy baby—unless the mother herself is infected with the pox—is for the birth mother to nurse the child. Eutrapelus is unequivocal on the topic.

This brings me to a related colloquy, "A Marriage in Name Only" ("Αγαμος γαμος sive Coniugium Impar"). The two interlocutors, Petronius and Gabriel, vent their anger against the parents of Iphigenia, described as in the flower of youth, who has been wed to Pompilius Blenus, known for two things, "lies, and the pox that doesn't yet have an exclusive name, since it goes by such a variety of them" (CWE, 40: 845).[19] To accentuate the injustice of the marriage, Gabriel describes the contrast between the "lovely" bride: "My clever Petronius, you have said she was some goddess: altogether lovely" and her ill-suited bridegroom: "Meanwhile, enter our handsome groom: nose broke, one foot dragging after the other (but less gracefully than the Swiss fashion would be), scurvy hands, a breath that would knock you over, lifeless eyes, head bound up, bloody matter exuding from nose and ears" (CWE, 40: 845). What Gabriel describes are the classic symptoms of syphilis: the pain in the joints causing the leg to drag, the rashes, foul breath, dazed eyes, and pus oozing from nose and ears. An anonymous poem of the sixteenth century refers to pieces of the nose falling off as a result of the disease.[20] The reader feels the anger of the two interlocutors against the parents for ignoring the well-being of their daughter for the sake of having a knight in the family.

> GABRIEL: To my way of thinking this treatment is more cruel than flinging her naked to the bears, or lions, or crocodiles. (CWE, 40: 845)
> PETRONIUS: If I had a one-eyed daughter who was lame in the bargain and as deformed as Homer's Thersites was, and dowerless to boot, I would refuse a son-in-law of that sort. (CWE, 40: 846)

Gabriel goes on to describe the stages of syphilis: "Yet this plague is both more hideous and more harmful than every kind of leprosy for it progresses quickly, recurs over and over again, and often kills, while leprosy sometimes allows a man to live to a ripe old age" (CWE, 40: 846). Having dismissed as false the excuse that her parents were ignorant of the bridegroom's infection, Gabriel runs down the list of the man's vices: gaming, drinking, prodigality, lying. Setting up Gabriel to divulge the true reason for the parents' pursuing the marriage, Petronius asks innocently: "Still, there must be something to recommend him to her parents." Gabriel replies ironically: "Only the glorious title of knight" (CWE, 40: 846). Petronius points out the contradiction in that a knight is meant for the saddle, but this knight's pox "scarcely allows him to sit in the saddle" (846).

The fault lies not with the girl but with the parents, whose responsibility it is to sanction a harmonious union. Like Rabelais and Marguerite de Navarre, Erasmus expounds through his interlocutors that the parents must pursue a suitable union for their children. Rabelais's Gargantua accepts his role in ensuring that his son, the prince Pantagruel, find a suitable mate; Marguerite de Navarre's narrator Parlamente, as well as the protagonist of the twenty-first tale of the *Heptaméron* herself, Rolandine, blame both her father and the queen (in the mother's absence) for failing to pursue a suitable marriage for Rolandine.[21] Renier Leushuis comments that Erasmus viewed marriage not as *mysterium* but as *sacramentum*— as a "symbolic representation of the divine mysteries" (Leushuis, 1285). Since it is a symbolic representation of the *mysterium* and not a mystery itself, it is dissoluble (Leushuis, 1286). For Erasmus, "the sacrament was foremost a sign of *amicitia,* and the marital bond a mystical joining of two souls in one reminiscent of the classical male *philia,* an aspect that no theologian before him had stressed so aggressively" (1286). This bond of "harmonious friendship" is far from the image of Iphigenia's unfortunate union with the pox-ridden knight.

Gabriel represents the Erasmian viewpoint that an unjust marriage can be annulled: "But if she married the baneful pest when he misrepresented himself as sound—if I were pope I'd annul this marriage even if it had been made with a thousand marriage contracts" (CWE, 40: 851). Petronius echoes the orthodox Catholic view: "On what pretext, since a marriage lawfully contracted cannot be annulled by mortal man?" (851). Gabriel responds with the example of legal annulment where a slave marries a maid under the pretext that he is a freeman (851). The issue is the survival of the marriage structure and the ability of the couple to procreate. Sexual relations between the syphilitic husband and Iphigenia would threaten both her health and the health of any unborn child. The only suitable remedy for her dilemma is to annul the marriage, a solution that partially repairs the injustice done her by the knight and her parents. In the immediate future, she is best to "cover her mouth with her hand when her husband kisses her and [to] sleep with him armed" (CWE, 40: 854). The long-term solution for the epidemic itself is to quarantine those infected by the pox. There follows a discussion of sacrificing the happiness of a few for the common good—something done in Italy during outbreaks of the plague (853). Both interlocutors have an awareness that the pox is more dangerous than the plague:

> Yet how much less is the peril from plague than from the pox! Rarely does the plague affect close relatives; as a rule it spares the aged; and those it does attack it either releases quickly or returns to health stronger than ever. *This* disease is simply slow but sure death, or rather burial. Victims are wrapped like corpses in cloths and unguents. (CWE, 40: 853)

The colloquy ends with one of several ironic comments, one that underscores the Erasmian use of Lucian's dialogical model and yet stresses the fatal blow dealt by the pox to the family structure. Petronius had been dispatched to write an epithalamium for the couple but will instead compose an epitaph for them. The ironic conclusion of the colloquy alerts the reader to the very serious threat posed by the epidemic in a time when religious and military conflict demands the mobilization of Europe's population. With families willing to trade the health and happiness of their daughters for the acquisition of titles, the Erasmian concept of marriage as an affectionate and holy joining of minds and bodies, as he expounds in *The Praise of Marriage,* is imperiled: "For what is sweeter than living with a woman with whom you are most intimately joined not merely by the bonds of affection but by physical union as well."[22] In the colloquy "Coniugium" ("Marriage"), Eulalia states "a wife must take every precaution to be pleasing to her husband in sexual relations, in order that married love may be rekindled and renewed and any annoyance or boredom driven out of mind" (CWE, 39: 318). It is clear that both the mind and body are engaged in the marriage enterprise.

While the integrity of marriage is first and foremost the subject of this colloquy, Petronius and Gabriel come up with a few ways to try to fend off the pox. First, they suggest that only one's personal barber should shave an individual; second, that one should wear the sort of mask worn by alchemists—with glasses to block the eyes and an opening over the mouth and nostrils to limit the intake of noxious air; third, that no one shall be both a barber and a surgeon; fourth, that only husbands and wives sleep in the same bed; and finally, back to the topic of inns mentioned earlier, that sheets be changed between guests (CWE, 40: 853). These are simple remedies that if adopted would greatly improve the standards of hygiene.

Discussion of the pox embraces a larger world picture than personal and communal hygiene. It is connected throughout the *Colloquies* with a broader picture of conflict in Europe and beyond. Erasmus and his interlocutors seem to acknowledge Charles V's responsibility for expansionism and provocation of his neighbors, as will be recalled from Eutrapelus's comment that "Charles is preparing to extend the boundaries of his realm" ("The New Mother," CWE, 39: 592). There seems to be sympathy for François I, detained in Spain by the Spanish, and hope that the rulers of Europe will come to a truce. Yet a second source of conflict comes from the churches and the parishioners in their care: "The peasants raise dangerous riots and are not swayed from their purpose, despite so many massacres. The commons are bent on anarchy; the church is shaken to its very foundations by menacing factions. On every side the seamless coat of Jesus is torn to shreds" (CWE, 39: 592). This comment, made so early in the evangelical reform, was echoed by Protestants and Catholics alike throughout the century as the atrocities committed in the name of religion multiplied.

In the colloquy "Ιχθυοφαγια" ("A Fish Diet"), there is a call from the Salt-Fishmonger for a truce. Peace is, in fact, according to Bierlaire, a major theme of not just this colloquy but of the *Colloquies* in general. Erasmus was obsessed with the theme of peace throughout his life: "Le thème de la paix, qui a hanté la conscience d'Érasme durant toute sa vie, est un des thèmes majeurs des *Colloques,* oeuvre de sa vie" (Bierlaire, *Les Colloques,* 181). If the fishmonger were emperor, he would call for "agreement without delay with the king of France." Were he emperor, he would try to create peace with the king of France and give him his liberty: "I grant you life and liberty. I accept you as an ally instead of an enemy" (CWE, 40: 688). The clemency would win over more friends than all the battles and conquests that have taken place.[23] The butcher agrees: "Certainly France, nay the whole world, might thus be bound in friendship" (CWE, 40: 689). It is at this point that the butcher uses a metaphor that will become commonplace in the second half of the sixteenth century—the use of the syphilitic sore or ulcer, this new pandemic, as a metaphor for the civil and religious conflict plaguing Europe and spilling over into the New World. The butcher adds: "For if this sore is covered up by bad terms rather than truly healed, I fear that when the wound is opened on some occasion soon afterwards, the old poison may burst out with more harm than ever" (CWE, 40: 689).[24] Remember that the Carthusian had accused the soldier of bringing back an ulcerated soul to his wife and family as a result of his frequenting prostitutes while away at war (CWE, 39:335). This ulcer threatens Europe's body and soul.

In an oblique fashion, the interlocutors associate the subjects of peace and health. By pursuing peace for the people's and Christ's sake and by treating enemies with clemency, both Charles V and the Pope would create a model for the Christian world: "This would truly cure the prejudice against the papal name and bring real and lasting glory" (CWE, 40: 689). The people of the world would no longer suffer at the hands of ambitious political and religious leaders. If religious leaders acted only for the "glory of Christ and the salvation of mankind," world order would be restored, for there would be no need for factions nor for personal or national ambition (689). "The Fish Diet" targets laws having to do with diet and health, such as those mandating days of fasting and feasting, arguing that it is best to follow nature's law—the same law that mothers should follow when caring for their babies. Conflict over dietary laws is among the laws likely to cause conflict and factionalism—especially regarding the interdiction of certain game and seafood. In the words of the fish monger: "Therefore I should think that the law which Nature herself also gave, and which is perpetual and inviolable, ought to be held more authoritative than the one that did not always exist and was later to be abrogated" (CWE, 40: 684). Nature trumps dietary laws imposed by religious sects, which are subject to change and human error.

Toward the end of the dialogue, the fishmonger expands the notion of nature to include the oversight of the health of mind and body: "Whatever Christ ordained, he ordained for the health of body and mind. Nor does any pope arrogate so much power to himself that by his regulations he would force anyone to risk his life; for example, by evening fasting a man gets insomnia and the insomnia causes delirium, he is a self-murderer, contrary both to the intention of the church and to the will of God" (CWE, 40: 712). Franz Bierlaire suggests that Erasmus engages civic-minded people to seek moderation that protects both liberty and the public good. Such moderation is to everyone's advantage and favors not just those in power—whether princes or men of the cloth (Bierlaire, *Érasme et ses Colloques*, 90).

Christ looks to maintaining people's physical and mental health, and so moderation in the observation of such laws should be encouraged to preserve the health of humankind.[25] The excesses of war and expansionism—the first a consequence of the second—have led to the outbreak of the pox and to the spread of the dreaded disease. As Marjorie O'Rourke Boyle has pointed out, Erasmus makes a clear analogy between the human body and the body politic. She cites Erasmus's letter to Henry VIII, on dedicating his *Peraphrases in evangelium Lucae* to the British monarch. In advising Henry VIII to abandon his alliance with Charles V against Francis I, Erasmus states: "The republic is a kind of body . . . Its pestilences and diseases are evil mores."[26] War was a "scourge to the already broken body of the Christian nations" (Boyle, 163). Although the disease has already been unleashed in Europe, at least peace and clemency can restore Europe to its earlier order, where young men can resume their rightful place with their families rather than roaming across the countryside of Europe, where they pillage, plunder, and spread the pox. The social structure that is at the base of civic life—the family—will be restored and maintained so that the health of young men and their wives and children will not be threatened. That the recipe to restore world order issues from the mouths of a fishmonger and a butcher demonstrates Erasmus's faith in the resilience of the human spirit and his Evangelical belief that common sense is not the product of erudition.[27]

3

Cannibalism and Syphilis in the Context of Religious Controversy

THE OUTBREAK of syphilis in the Old World followed closely the return of Columbus's crew to Europe. The virulence of the epidemic took hold of the physicians and the less-schooled and more practical surgeons in their quest for an efficacious remedy. In turn, as the epidemic spread, textual and visual representations of suffering syphilitics became rooted in the literary works of sixteenth-century humanists. From the outset, explorers, cosmographers, and missionaries had connected syphilis with sexual activity in the same indigenous people who were known for the practice of cannibalism. As I have pointed out elsewhere, it was a widely held belief that syphilis was connected with cannibalism, and was retribution for the unnatural act of eating one's own kind.[1] What I will endeavor to show in this chapter is that syphilis and cannibalism—markers of the exploration of the New World—became signs for exploring the thornier issues of religious controversy in the Old World. Protestants and Catholics—whether physicians, literary figures, or theologians—explored syphilis and its connection to the exploration of the New World to serve their own professional, religious, and political causes.

The cosmographer and former Franciscan André Thevet informs us in his work, *Histoire de deux voyages* (1587–88), that he subscribed to the theory of the American origin of syphilis. He states that the "la maladie des Pians" had as its root cause not climate or foul air in the region, but the libidinous inclinations of the women, always eager to seek sexual relations with their husbands: "Car ce people, comme il est brutal, est fort addonné à la paillardise, et sur tout les femmes, lesquelles cerchent, et pratiquent tous les moyens qu'elles peuvent à esmouvoir leurs mari" [For this people, in consequence of its animal nature, is very much given to lecherous behavior, and especially the women who seek and practice all ways to arouse their husbands].[2] He goes on to make the link between this venereal disease, probably yaws, and syphilis:[3]

> Qui me fait penser . . . que de cette malversation, et compagnie avec ces femmes ainsy eschauffées, cette maladie a pris sa source, et n'est autre chose que cette belle verole, laquelle est à present si espanduë en toute la Chrestienté, qu'il n'est plus saison de l'appeller mal de Naples, ou mal francois, ains le mal commun de tout le monde.
>
> Which makes me think . . . that from this lewd conduct and relationships with these hotblooded women the illness took its origins and is no other than the fair pox, which is now so spread through all of Christendom that it is no longer appropriate to call it the Naples illness or the French disease but a world-wide disease. (Thevet, 211)

Now one might ask what Thevet's remarks have to do with the Wars of Religion waging in France. His *Histoire* is actually a rewriting and elaboration of his earlier work, *Les Singularitez de la France Antarctique, autrement nommée Amerique: & de plusieurs Terres et Isles decouvertes de nostre temps* (1557–58) and of passages from the *Cosmographie universelle* (1575). The ill-fated expedition of Nicolas de Villegagnon gave birth to a notable rivalry between two travelers—the Franciscan/cosmographer who would serve Catherine de Médici through her sons François II, Charles IX, and Henri III, and the Calvinist follower and later pastor Jean de Léry. Both had been participants in the expedition of Villegagnon—Thevet as chaplain and subsequently Léry, who claims that Villegagnon had written to Geneva asking the Reformed Church "non seulement que on luy envoyast des Ministres de la parole de Dieu: mais aussi pour tant mieux reformer luy et ses gens, et mesme pour attirer les sauvages à la cognoissance de leur salut, que quelques nombres d'autres personages bien instruits en la Religion Chrestienne accompagnassent lesdits Ministres" [to send him not only ministers of the Word of God, but also to send a number of other persons well instructed in the Christian religion to accompany the ministers, the better to reform him and his people, and even to bring the savages to the knowledge of their salvation].[4] Léry explains that although he returned to France from Brazil in 1558 and had shown to others the "memoires que j'avois, la pluspart escrits d'ancre de Bresil, et en l'Amerique mesme" [memoirs, most of them written with brazilwood ink, and in America itself], he had no intention of proceeding to publication. It is only when faced with repeated factual errors about Brazil to be found in Thevet's *Cosmographie* that he felt compelled to write to correct the errors and to put straight the libelous accusations against the ministers of the Reformed Church and those who accompanied them at Villegagnon's request: "À fin, di-je, de repousser ces impostures de Thevet, j'ay esté comme contraint de mettre en lumière tout le discours de nostre voyage" (63/xlvi) [Therefore, in order to refute these falsehoods of Thevet, I have been compelled to set forth a complete report of our voyage].

The Tupi, an indigenous people of Brazil, were pulled unwittingly into the French Wars of Religion in the wake of the violence of the St. Bartholomew's Day Massacre as a consequence of these accounts of their cultural practices. Léry, like his fellow Frenchman Thevet, observes the "maladie incurable qu'ils [the Tupi people] nomment *Pians*" (469/173) [the incurable disease that they call *pians*]. Léry for once agrees with the judgment of Thevet that the disease is transmitted sexually—that it is the consequence of "paillardise," lechery. Yet, ever the patient observer and careful recorder of details, he comments that he has observed children afflicted with *pians*. Léry's notation would be one of the early observations that venereal diseases, including syphilis, can be transmitted to the children, something that European physicians and surgeons began to record: "Laquelle [pians] combine qu'ordinairement elle se prenne et provienne de paillardise, j'ay neantmoins veu avoir à de jeunes enfans qui en estoyent aussi couverts, qu'on en voit par deçà de la petite verole" (469/172) [Ordinarily, it is a result of lechery, but I have also seen it in young children, who were covered all over with it just as children over here are afflicted with smallpox]. His description of the open sores mirrors the descriptions of European medical specialists treating the syphilis: "Pustules plus larges que le pouce, lesquelles s'espandent par tout le corps et jusques au visage: ceux qui en sont entachez en portent aussi bien les marques toute leur vie, que font les verolez et chancreux de par deçà, de leur turpitude et vilenie" (469/172) [Pustules as wide as a thumb, which spread over the entire body, even to the face, so that those who are spotted with it carry the marks of their turpitude and baseness all through their lives, just as our pox-ridden folk do over here]. Writing in 1579, the renowned physician Jean Fernel speaks of the appearance of the "postules" in the earlier years of the outbreak: countless, protruding, comparable in form and size to acorns ("sans nombre," "saillantes," "comparables pour la forme et la grandeur à des glands de chêne").[5]

It is the vividness of Léry's depiction of the sores and the physical signs of the disease that strike the reader as well as Léry's and Thevet's recognition that this was a global epidemic that infected the indigenous people of the New World and inhabitants of the Old World alike. The common link is lecherous behavior—noted in Léry's description of the interpreter, "natif de Rouen, lequel s'estant veautré en toutes sortes de paillardises parmi les femmes et filles sauvages, en avoit si bien recue son salaire, que son corps et son visage estans aussi couverts et deffigurez de ces *Pians* que s'il eust esté vray ladre, les places y estoyent tellement imprimées, qu' impossible luy fut de jamais les effacer" (*Histoire*, 469/172–73) [a native of Rouen, who had wallowed in all sorts of lechery with the savage women and girls, and so truly received the ways of his sins that his body and face were as disfigured by these *pians* as if he had been a leper; the marks were so deeply imprinted that they could never be effaced].

Léry's description of the disputes between the Calvinist ministers and Villegagnon's men, Catholics who continue to hold to the literal rather than the figurative meaning of the transformation of the Eucharist into the body and blood of Christ, leads to blending the image of cannibalism with the theory of transubstantiation: "Ils vouloyent neantmoins non seulement grossierement, plustost que spirituellement, manger la chair de Jesus Christ, mais qui pis estoit, à la maniere des sauvages nommez Ou-ëtacas . . . ils la vouloeyent mascher et avaler toute crue" (*Histoire*, 177/41) [They wanted not only to eat the flesh of Jesus Christ grossly rather than spiritually, but what was worse, like the savages named *Ouetaca*, . . . they wanted to chew and swallow it raw]. The Papists, including the turncoat Villegagnon, are guilty of spiritual cannibalism. Their practices are classed with the lecherous eating habits and sexual conduct of the indigenous peoples of the New World. Léry follows this last description with a portrait of Villegagnon, and this portrait reveals an irony worthy of Rabelais or Bonaventure Des Périers: "Toutesfois Villegagnon faisant tousjours bonne mine, et protestant ne desirer rien plus que d'estre droitement enseigné" (*Histoire*, 177/41) [However, Villegagnon, still putting on a fair countenance and protesting that he desired nothing more than to be rightly instructed].

Edicts published and disseminated in French towns ordering individuals afflicted with the pox or "grosse vérole" to leave the confines of Paris are found in the archives from 1497.[6] To examine how the pox or "grosse vérole" is linked to religious conflict between Catholics and Protestants, I will examine literary texts in which the pox is juxtaposed with references to religious controversy. Let me begin with a satirical poem, "La Pastenostre des Verollez, avec une complaincte contre les medecins," published as a four-leaf booklet, date and author unspecified. Its tone, spelling, images, and ironic juxtaposition of bawdy vernacular verse with Latin phrases from the Mass recall the Evangelical Reformist works of Rabelais, Marot, and Bonaventure des Périers, and the time period specified by Montaiglon supports this.[7]

Linking the "Our Father"—the Pater Noster—to the plight of the *vérolé* is at once audacious and satirical in its vivid description of the physical symptoms of syphilis within a context of forgiveness and deliverance from evil.

> *Pater noster*, très glorieux,
> Nostre Saulveur, comme je croy,
> N'oublie pas les veroleux
> Qui dressent leur prière à toy,
>   *Qui es in coelis*
> (Montaiglon, I, 68)
>
> *Our Father*, full of glory
> Our Savior, as I believe,
> Do not forget the poxy ones
> Who raise their prayers to you
>   *Who art in Heaven*

The first four lines of each stanza evoke the plight of the syphilitic, and the fourth line is a Latin verse from the Pater Noster—heightening the comic effect since the audience anticipates the Latin phrase, here used in an ironic context of syphilis. The poet paints a forgiving Father more intent on listening than the physicians who "ne voyent goutte" [don't see (i.e., understand) anything] and who milk their clients, "et ne nous laissent ung denier" [and don't leave us a farthing] (68). The direct, intimate discourse between believer and creator is reminiscent of the healing power of the Lord, the image of the Christus medicus depicted in the works of poets and storytellers with Evangelical leanings.[8] Early Evangelical humanism, whether stressing reform within the church or in a break from the church, stressed the healing power of Christ in terms of the body and the soul. Rudolph Arbesmann explains that Saint Augustine returned more than forty times in his sermons to the metaphor of the Christus medicus to illustrate the concept of redemption.[9] By humbling himself, Christ came down to earth to save humankind. Pride had caused the fall, and it is through Christ's humility that the sin of pride will be forgiven. Christ heals both the body and soul, but "only the humble soul is capable of following Christ," a concept taught by Saint Paul (Arbesmann, 9). In this parody of the Pater Noster, the syphilitic bypasses worldly physicians to entreat ("Je te supplie très humblement") the divine physician to heal both body and soul. The symptoms of the pox—ill temper, cankers, scabies, and gout—are indeed the "bitter medicine" with which the lowly sufferers of the pox will prepare themselves for possible redemption. John Henderson cites the Medieval Dominican Domenica Cavalca's reference to the "corporeal sufferings of Christ" as a "bitter medicine" taken to redeem the sin of humankind (Henderson, 115).

> Mais tu t'en ris et nous escouttes,
> Et nous souffrons en ce martyre
> (Des) regnes, chancres, gales et gouttes,
> Tant qu'en la fin nous fauldra dire:
> *Fiat voluntas tua*
> (Montaiglon, I, 69)

> But you make light [of our predicament] and listen to us,
> And we suffer this affliction
> Bouts of ill temper, cankers, scabies and gout
> So finally we must say
> *Let thy will be done*

As the patients appealed to doctors and surgeons for a remedy, so the syphilitic of this poem looks to the heavenly Father for relief:

> Si tu as point quelque oignement
> Pour nous bien guerir et soubdain
> Je te supplie très humblement
> Que n'actendes point à demain;
> *Da nobis hodie*
> (Montaiglon, I, 70)

> If you happen to have an ointment
> To cure us quickly and fully
> I humbly beg you not to wait for tomorrow
>> But to give it to us today

The mention of therapeutic ointments brings to mind the image of the *vérolez* depicted in the prologue of *Pantagruel*, mentioned earlier in this book. He evokes both the mercury-based ointments rubbed on the bodies of the syphilitics and the shivers and pains they endured: the "well greased" face ("le visaige leur reluyssoit") and the "chattering" teeth ("les dentz leurs tressailloyent").[10]

I remarked in chapter 1 that Rabelais bids those afflicted with the pox to listen to the reading of "quelque page" of *Pantagruel* to allay the pains of the disease, much as women in childbirth listen to "la vie de saincte Marguerite" [the Life of Saint Margaret] (*Pantagruel*, 215/134). In the same facetious tone, the narrator goes on to say that his *Chronicque Gargantuine* has sold more books in two months than the Bible in nine years ("car il en a esté plus vendu par les imprimeurs en deux moys qu'il ne sera acheté de Bibles en neuf ans"; 216/13). I recognize the setting of Evangelical humanism so common to Erasmus, Bonaventure Des Périers, and Marguerite de Navarre in the gentle and ironic chiding of those who address the saints, such as Saint Margaret, instead of putting their trust directly in God. Like the "Patenostre des Verollez," Rabelais is not averse to linking spiritual and temporal concerns: prayers and pox, Bibles and commerce.

Echoing the anonymous author of the "Patenostre des Verollez," the narrator of Rabelais's 1552 prologue to the *Quart Livre* prays for the syphilitics' return to good health. He counsels them to wait with patience and faith that "s' il plaist au bon Dieu" health will be restored (581/435). It is a return to health based on keeping modest goals, humbling oneself before God, recognizing one's imperfections—and limiting one's discussion of the power and predestination of God's will: "la puissance et praedestination de Dieu" (581). These are all themes that form a part of the Evangelical humanist doctrine. Earlier in the same prologue, Rabelais appeals to good health ("Santé") through the intermediary of Christ ("avecques l'ayde du benoist Servateur"; 568/426), a reference to the healing power of "the blessed Savior." Within the same context, he returns to a favorite example of Augustine's, the modest and humble wish of the small but wealthy tax collector Zaccheus to see Christ by climbing a tree. Appreciating his humble act of faith, Christ goes to the home of

Zaccheus, who upon welcoming Jesus, vows to restore fourfold anything he has taken illegally. It is here that Jesus speaks of salvation coming to a son of Abraham—the healing of the tax collector's sins through his faith in the Lord (Luke 19:1–10; Arbesmann, 16).

As Bakhtin has pointed out, Rabelais turns to the "bas corporel"—lower extremities—to invoke the laughter of the carnival in opposition to the hypocritical position of the Parisian theologians regarding procreation and bodily functions. Gout and syphilis—diseases of excess—are "joyeuses maladies" [happy diseases], discussion of which leads to ecclesiastical censureship—"a lie directed against the gay truth" of men's and women's sexual organs.[11] Rabelais's narrator urges his poxy ones to ask for health—a modest wish: "Humiliez vous davant sa sacrée face et recongnoissez vos imperfections" (581/435) [Humble yourselves before His holy face, and recognize your imperfections]. His favored readers, the "goutteux"/"verolez," have a strong faith that is lacking in the elevated discourse of the Sorbonne faculty, and so based on such humility, and if the good Lord is willing ("s'il plaist au bon Dieu"), health should be granted these humble sufferers ("vous obtiendrez santé"; 581/435).

Reminiscent of the facetious tone and popular origins of the "Pastenostre des verollez," published in the same collection by Montaiglon, is the "Sept marchans de Naples," author unknown. The commercial setting in a market evokes the public backdrop of many of the *contes* and *nouvelles* of the first half of the sixteenth century, such as may be seen in Du Fail's *Propos rustiques*. As Montaiglon states, the seven "marchans" are not sellers but buyers one and all: a soldier, a monk, a student, a blind man, a villager, a merchant, and a pleasure seeker or "bragard."[12] They have all "bought" the pox or "mal de Naples" through the normal means of transmission: "Pour ung plaisir, mille douleurs" (Montaiglon, II, 110–11) [For one pleasure, a thousand pains]. The poem captures the ubiquitous nature of syphilis and its rapid spread through all social classes.

The tone is light in spite of the depiction of suffering by the afflicted, who bear many symptoms of the disease: deformity, inflamed facial and bodily sores, yellow teeth, painful joints, swollen members. The poem unfolds as a chronicle of the spread of the disease. I have spoken of the transmission of the disease from the sailors and adventurers accompanying Columbus to the New World to the invading French soldiers and mercenaries, whose presence in Naples gave rise to the two appellations: *le mal français (morbus gallicus)* and *le mal de Naples*. It is noteworthy that the mercenary soldier is the first to speak, given that soldiers were key to spreading the disease among the camp followers in Italy: "Marchant je fuz, et, sans bailler, grand erre / On me vendit un dangereux caterre, / Lequel on dit la maladye de Naples" (Montaiglon 99) [Client was I, and without paying, swiftly / I was sold a dangerous illness, / Which is called the sickness of Naples]. The mercenary calls to mind his Erasmian counterpart in the colloquy between the soldier and the Carthusian, when the monk points out that among the prizes the soldier brings back is the pox (CWE, 39: 335).

In the facetious anticlerical but not bitter tone of the era, the work describes how the monk, against the orders of his religious community, relished amorous pleasure, and instead of roses, reaped red sores for his activities: "Car on deffend, en tout temps et saison, / Le marchander à tout bon religieux. / . . . Et, comme fol, trenchant de l'amoureux, / Pour un plaisir, alors bien savoureux, / En lieu de roses j'achapté des boutons" (Montaiglon, II: 101). The bawdy language in the vein of Rabelais is notable as the monk speaks of lusting after a transaction made between two good hams ("un marché fis entre deux beaulx jambons"; 101). Common to the symbolic language of sixteenth-century tales, he mentions exchanging love's pleasures for creams and pains in the monk's dormitory ("Je suis en dortoir, / Sans plaisir avoir, / Criant, jour et nuyt"), his pastoral staff for a crutch: "En lieu de crosse ou baston pastoral / Il me convient porter une quinette" (102).

In targeting itinerant people, soldiers, students, and pleasure seekers who come in contact daily with new people in the public streets and markets, the poet accurately depicts the spread of communicative diseases. Again, his student ("escollier") mirrors Rabelais's *écolier limousin*, as Montaiglon points out (II: 103, n. 1). For his money ("ung beau grant blanc"), he has received more than he bargained for ("On me bailla sur-le-champ tout comptant"): aches and pains in the joints ("J'ay les gouttes qui me tourmentent tant"; 104). The same transformation is witnessed in the pleasure seeker, who trades his light step and handsome mien for swollen feet ("En mes jambes les gouttes sont enflées"; 108). Reference is made to the necessity of concealing the infected private parts and excretions beneath elaborate boots, breaches, and codpiece: "Mais pour couvrir la brague, raison briefve, / Des brodequins je porte par dessus, A celle fin que, s'aulcune s'enliève, / Ou aultrement, pour bien purger (mon pus), / Tout est couvert, et on n'en parle plus" (108–109). Unseemly pus was not only repellent to the ladies but might lead to expulsion from the urban areas from which sufferers of the pox were banned, as evidenced in the edicts such as the Arrêt de Parlement of Paris dating from as early as 1497 (Harrison 6).

In his *Propos rustiques* (1547), Noël du Fail follows in Rabelais's tradition of viewing "la belle verole" as a happy disease. Anselme, one of his devisants, recounts the tale of the spendthrift Tailleboudin, who goes through his inheritance in less time than it took Panurge to go through the revenue given him by Pantagruel to run the castle of Salmagundi (*Le Tiers Livre,* chapter 3). Running against the thematics of the *Propos Rustiques*—the glories of the village life—Tailleboudin extols the virtues of the urban community of beggars (*mauvais garçons* or *coquillards*) because of the money they can make feigning to be blind, mute, or afflicted with leprosy. Tailleboudin is himself in possession of few material objects: dice, cards, a tennis racquet, and a box full of ointment for curing his pox ("une Boette pleine d'onguens pour guerir son chancre").[13] He and his fellow "gueux" live off the generosity of those pilgrims who believe in miracles and pay them generously as "blind" or "deaf" vagabonds on the streets. The same pilgrims are amazed to see the efficacy of their alms giving, when, on the "rue des Miracles" in Bourges, the blind sees and the leper suddenly is cured. Tailleboudin ends his eulogy of the joys of begging with the story of a partnership with a young woman who pretends to be his virgin daughter. He ends up selling her to "un gros chanoine," taking her back, and reselling her to "plus de quinze, qui tous eurent la verole" (105) [more than fifteen who all are infected with the pox]. Du Fail's skepticism regarding "good works" and pilgrimages reveals his analytic perspective as a lawyer and his evangelical humanism.[14] These traits come through in his view of syphilis as a disease of those who balance the desires of body and soul and flee doctrines that deny the procreative impulses of men and women. This positive perspective would change as the persecution of evangelical preachers heated up and the violence of the Wars of Religion grew. Syphilis and its root cause, lascivious behavior or "paillardise," took on a more sinister role in becoming a rhetorical weapon in theological and civil discord on both the Protestant and Catholic sides of the controversy.

The Protestant satirical work *Satyres chrestiennes de la cuisine papale* (1560), thought by Eugénie Droz and Charles-Antoine Chamay to be authored by Théodore de Bèze, attacks the moral depravity of the priests, cardinals, and Pope as he depicts them in an enormous papal kitchen—seat of all excess and moral decadence.[15] In making his point about the hypocrisy of the Catholic administrators, the narrator/poet depicts the former president of the Parlement de Paris, Pierre Lizet, as the syphilitic he was at the time he banned many Protestants, including Bèze, for heresy: "Quoy plus? Nos Maistres sorbonniers / aussi luisans'qu'une lanterne

/ Sont au milieu de la taverne" (47, vv. 159–161) [What else? Our Sorbonne professors / As shiny as a lantern / Are gathered in the tavern]. The shine refers not only to Lizet's *nez de vérolé*, already immortalized in an anonymous poem, "la Complainte de Messire Pierre Liset sur le trespas de son feu nez"—perhaps by Bèze himself—but also to the ointments used to treat syphilis, by which other *Maistres sorbonniers* were also afflicted.

In the *Satyres*, the nose becomes a leitmotif for clerical hypocrisy and licentious behavior, as a vaguely disguised Lizet reappears as Messire Niçaise, a member of the colloquium presiding over the end of the *Satyres*. In a delightful play—if indeed Théodore de Bèze is author of both the *Complainte* and the *Satyres*—Messire Niçaise evokes the poem depicting the loss of the nose: "Avez-vous point ouy nouvelle / D'une risee solennelle / Qu'a fait de son nez trespassé / . . . Un certain poëte à demy" (160, vv. 357–61) [Haven't you heard about / The grave mocking piece / About the loss of a nose / Made by an amateur poet]. The *Complainte de Messire Pierre Liset sur le trespas de son feu nez* begins by mentioning the syphilitic pustules on Messire Pierre's nose: "Messire Pierre estonné / De voir son nez boutonné / Prest à tomber par fortune / De la vérole importune" ("Complainte," *Satyres Chrestiennes de la Cuisine papale,* 162–63) [Sir Peter surprised / To see his pock-marked nose / Ready to fall as luck would have it / Of the troublesome pox].

Instead of attributing the lascivious ways to the cannibals, as Thevet and Léry would do, it is now the Catholic clergy at all ranks—monks, priests, cardinals, and Pope—who are faulted for their degeneracy. Notable is the attack on the interaction between clergy and the "beguines"—those often widowed ladies who retired to the quiet life of the convent and gave themselves to weaving, spinning, embroidering, and doing laundry to meet the needs of the clergy: "LECTEUR, escoute un autre vice / Ces couvents du monde retraits, / Sont de ce manoir les retraits, / Et cuvier à buer les linges / De ces singesses [les beguines] et singes [moines/clergé]" (*Satyre IIII*, 73, vv. 1–5) [READER, listen for another vice / These convents withdrawn from the world, / Are the latrines of this manor house, / And laundry tub for dirty clothes / Of these female and male monkeys]. The poet plays on the words for "lascivious" (*lascive*) and "laundry" (*lescive*) in underscoring the wanton behavior of the inhabitants of the convent: "L'orgueil d'Aman, et la luxure / Soit en evesché ou en cure, / Vuident, et de façon lascive / Espanchent en bas la lescive" (*Satyre IIII*, 74, vv. 20–23) [The pride of Aman and immoral behavior / Whether in the bishopric or parsonage, / Take hold and in a wanton manner / Spread down the washing]. In calling on a fictive reader ("LECTEUR") to listen to yet another vice attributed to the Catholics, the narrator engages the listener in a humorous game of words (with "washing" and "wanton" alongside "retraits," evoking both latrines and convents). Antonia Szabari reminds us of the distinct rhetorical stance of the reformed authors, who actively engaged their readers in a "community of laughter" (*Less Rightly Said*, 121).

It is here that the description of gastronomic indulgence links back to cannibalism and the religious controversy that led the Protestants to accuse the Catholics of anthropophagy both in the Old World and in the New. In *Satyre V*, "Banquet Papal," the poet/narrator evokes the Catholic clergy's consumption of the body of Christ: "Mieux vous vaudroit, Anthropophages, / Pis il y a, ô Theophages, / Que pour vostre dernier renfort / Vous mangez Dieu comme un refort" (*Satyre V*, 103, vv. 384–87) [Better for you, Cannibals / Even worse, O God Eaters / That for your last rations / You eat God as one might horseradish.] No doubt the white of the horseradish is compared to the white of the host. Szabari notes that in the papal kitchen, "theological error" has transformed the communion host into the "god of white dough" (*Less Rightly Said*, 120). This papal banquet, earlier compared to a bed of fornication ("un lict de fornication"), is transformed into a literal feast of Christ's body—much as Léry and Thevet would describe the Tupis' vengeful act of consuming their enemy's flesh. The poet takes aim at the theory of transubstantiation—interpreting Christ's words literally: "Voyla comme Dieu vient sur terre / Pour estre avallé rustrement, / ou serré bien estroictement" (*Satyre V*, 109, vv. 489–91) [Here is how God comes to earth / To be swallowed crudely, / or held too tightly]. This poet, as Léry will do later, in reference to the Tupi, focuses on the act of swallowing the body of Christ. The reference to holding the host too tightly refers to the storing of the unused consecrated hosts between glass disks in a special cabinet over long periods of time, literally imprisoning God's body: "Mais le povre Dieu estourdi / Et de sa prison engourdi, / Ne va à pied ni à cheval / Ains de peur qu'il se face mal" (109, vv. 498–501) [But the poor, astonished God / And numb from his prison / Goes neither on foot or horseback / For fear of hurting himself]. The Protestant poet creates a comic image by pushing the literal interpretation of transubstantiation to its limits. As has been seen, Léry would accuse Villegagnon and his men of chewing and swallowing the body of Christ raw (*Histoire*, 177/41)—a similar extension of the doctrine of transubstantiation. As Frank Lestringant observes, the Tupinamba follow a more normal culinary process, in which the cannibals cook their enemies and then consume them, while the Catholic doctrine follows a "pre-Christian" and thus pagan process in which the cooked wafer is transformed into a raw body of Christ before ingestion—a process more savage than that of the indigenous people of Brazil.[16]

In the same year (1560) in which the *Satyres* appeared, Artus Désiré, eager to support the Catholic cause against the Protestant heresy, and in particular, against Clément Marot's French translation of the Psalms of David, composed and published the *Contrepoison des cinquante-deux chansons de Clément Marot*.[17] The title is important, in that it sets the religious controversy in the context of sickness of epidemic proportions. The depravity of the followers of the Reformed Church—which Désiré will portray in all its force—will only be stopped by the application of the appropriate remedy—the *contrepoison*—which he has concocted in his book. Marot's "chansons," falsely, Désiré claims, entitled "Psalmes," excite the unsuspecting souls of the faithful "à liberté, luxure et paillardise" (*Contrepoison*, A ii). Désiré evokes the same words, *luxure* and *paillardise,* to describe the licentious behavior of the Protestant clergy as Thevet and Léry had used to describe sexual degeneracy among the inhabitants of the New World. Perceived barbarism abroad has been brought home to recount the sexual excesses of Catholics and Protestants alike. Syphilis and its origins in the New World—shameless lasciviousness—have taken hold in the European mentality. Cannibalism, syphilis, and religious controversy are firmly intertwined.

Invoking the first words of Marot's translation for each psalm at the start of each *chanson,* Désiré appropriates from Marot the theme or image to begin his denunciation of Luther, Calvin, and their heretic followers: "Dans l'orde generation / De Luther plein d'abusion / Qui cerche sa concupiscence, / N'aura pas pour ayde et secours / A la fin de ses derniers iours" (*Contrepoison*, Chanson XX, 31) [In the sullied brood / Of Luther full of abuse / Who seeks lust / Will have no help or succor / At the end of his last days]. Schism and carnal behavior are one and the same to Désiré, as hypocrisy and lust had been for the Protestants like Bèze: "Les malheureux Schismatiques / Sont tant charnelz et lubriques / Et de si mauuais renom / Qu'ilz perdent par vaine gloire" (*Contrepoison*, Chanson XXXIIII, 50) [The wretched schismatic's / Are so wanton and lustful / And of such ill fame / That they lose by pride]. Heresy for Désiré, as for Thevet, is a form of epidemic—running wild as surely as syphilis continued to do through the sixteenth century: "Leur Heresie puante / est fluante / De sang de corruption, / Et par leur folle sotie / Est sortie / Toute ceste infection" (*Contrepoison,* Chanson XXVI, 40) [Their stinking Heresy runs rampant / With corrupted blood, / And out of their mad foolishness / Issues all this infection].[18] Désiré's use of " traditional theological notions and images," here seen in the words "heresy," "corruption," and "infection," used to refer to the contamination that comes through translation of the psalms into the vernacular, demonstrates Szabari's theory that the rhetoric of Catholic and Reformed polemicists is distinct. In opposition to the extreme wing of the Catholic Church represented by Désiré, the Reformed polemicists insist on the supremacy of scripture over all other forms of knowledge (Szabari, 8).

One poet who does not initially engage in the rhetoric of the pox is nonetheless dragged into the exchange of medical insults when he is accused of having the disease. It is not that Pierre de Ronsard is any less vitriolic in his attacks on Huguenot theology or its proponents, it is just that he generally eschews the couching of this bitter religious and civil conflict in terms of the pox.[19] He accuses the Huguenots of forgetting that the only weapons recommended by Saint Paul are humility, fasting, and tears: "Et saint Paul en preschant n'avoit pour toutes armes/Sinon l'humilité, les jeusnes et les larmes."[20] Addressing Catherine de Medici in "Continuation du discours des miseres de ce temps," he chastises the violence of attacks by the Reformed Church on the Catholic populace, and he accuses the Protestants of disobeying their king:

Et quoy? Brusler maisons, piller et brigander,
Tuer, assassiner, par force commander,
N'obeir plus aux Rois, amasser des armées,
Appellez-vous cela Eglises reformées?
(*Oeuvres complètes,* II: 551, vv. 8–11)

And what? Burning houses, pillaging and robbing,
Killing, assassinating, commanding by force,
No longer obeying our Kings, gathering armies,
Is that what you call the Reformed Churches?

While it is often the Huguenot preachers who claim to be the wronged party, those at the mercy of the highly armed soldiers of the Catholic army, Ronsard reverses the argument. In his "Response de Pierre de Ronsard aux injures et calomnies de je ne sçay quels predicantereaux et ministreaux de Genéve," he preaches charity and takes pity toward his accuser, frère Zamariel, the fictional incarnation of Antoine de la Roche-Chandieu, preacher and minister of the Reformed Church in Geneva.[21]

Ronsard speaks of his empathy toward "frère Zamariel," whom he saw starving ("descharné") and emaciated ("deshalé") in Paris. The poet depicts his compassion for the Huguenot preacher's tormented and sickly state ("Response aux injures," II: 601, v. 6). He suggests that Brother Zamariel, given his sickly appearance, is a much more likely candidate for the pox than he, for, in addition to the Huguenot's wretched appearance, he has been known for his amorous exploits: "Or, à ce qu'on disoit, ce mal tu avois pris / Travaillant au mestier de la belle Cypris" (II: 601, v. 11–12) [But, it was said that you had contracted this illness / Working the trade of the beautiful Cypris]. Cypris is a reference to Aphrodite. Despite the Huguenot's reputation for lovemaking "en divers lieux," the poet assumes a charitable attitude, befitting the king's chaplain that he is, and prays God to restore his sickly colleague to his former good health: "Je fis à Dieu priere / De te faire jouyr de ta santé premiere" (II: 601, vv. 17–18).[22]

Showing himself to be charitable and forgiving, Ronsard points out that the Huguenot preacher shows no such mercy to the poet, whom he accuses of having the pox: "Tu m'accuses, cafard, d'avoir la verolle" (II: 601, v. 21–22). Ronsard skillfully turns the charge of hypocrite, usually aimed at Catholic priests, to attack a Protestant minister. The poet reminds the Huguenot Zamariel that such a charge against Ronsard, court chaplain and poet, amounts to unbecoming and unsuitable behavior for one who purports to be a chaste preacher ("un chaste predicant"):

Un chaste predicant de faict et de parolle
Ne devroit jamais dire un propos si vilain;
Mais que sort-il du sac? cela dont il est plein.
Tousjours le volleur pense à la despouille prise,
Et tousjours le paillard parle de paillardise.
(II: 601)

A chaste preacher in deed and in speech
Should never utter such an ugly word;
But what does he take out of his sack? What it's full of.
The thief is always thinking of spoils taken,
And the lecher always speaks of filth.

That the Calvinist falls back on such filthy language only confirms Ronsard's later accusation that "Tu as en l'estomac un lexicon farci / De mots injurieux qui donnent à cognoistre / Que mechant escolier tu as eu mechant maistre" (II: 617, vv. 4–5) [You have in your gut a lexicon / Of scathing words that reveal / That as a lewd pupil you had a lewd teacher]. Ronsard cleverly demonstrates that the vices attributed to him by Zamariel/de la Roche-Chandieu are a reflection of the Huguenot's own failings. As proof, the poet cites his own healthy appearance and strong constitution ("mes nerfs bien tendus"/"taut nerves"; "mes veines bien fortes"/"sturdy veins"; 601, v. 34), in stark contrast to the emaciated look of the Huguenot preacher. That Ronsard is not tempted by the Protestant religion does not make him an atheist. In a bold series of statements, the poet collects evidence that the Huguenot's actions run counter to Christian and thus French concepts of justice: "Lequel est plus athée ou de moy ou de toy?" (II: 602, 16) [Which one is more atheist, you or me?].

Ronsard contrasts his own quiet obedience to the Crown ("En la loy du pays, en l'humble obeisance / Des Rois, des Magistrats" [II: 602, v. 18–19] [For the country's law in humbly obeying / Kings and Magistrates]) with the behavior of the Huguenot who has set the fury of the people against one another: "As fait que le voisin a tué son voisin, / Le pere son enfant, le cousin sons cousin?" (II: 602, 23–24) [Have put the neighbor to kill his neighbor / The father his child, the cousin his cousin?]. The most serious accusation from the poet is that the Huguenot preacher and his colleagues have twisted the meaning of the Gospels to suit their own personal interpretation, and in doing so, have misled innocent people:

> Qui fais de l'habile homme, et qui aux innocens
> Interpretes, malin, l'Evangile à ton sens;
> Qui as comme le brigand la Justice oppressée,
> Et sans-dessus-dessous la France renversée!
> (II: 602, 27–30)

> Who plays the clever man, and who interprets for the innocents,
> Deceitful person, the Gospel according to your own meaning;
> Who has, like a thief, overthrown Justice,
> And turned France upside down!

If, as Szabari suggests, the distinct rhetoric of reformed polemicists subordinates all writing and all knowledge to scripture, then here Ronsard turns Calvinist rhetoric against Zamariel by accusing the Huguenot preacher of having twisted the meaning of the Gospel to fit his individual interpretation: "Qui fais de l'habile homme, et qui aux innocens / Interpretes, malin, l'Evangile à ton sens" (Szabari, 8). Later in the same poem, Ronsard repeats this accusation of the Huguenot's tendency to distort the meaning of the Scriptures for theological purposes: "Tu as selon ton sens l'Evangile traitée" ("Response aux injures," II: 616, v. 32). The Catholic poet appropriates the language of his adversary to drive home the point.[23] The loser is France and its innocent people caught in the web of verbal and physical jousting, but through God's compassion for the "misères de l'homme," and through the actions of the queen mother and the young prince, Catherine de Medici and Charles IX, peace returns—an allusion to the Edict of Amboise in 1563, the year of the composition of the "Response aux injures et calomnies."

In the poem, Ronsard shifts the image of the pox, a disease the Huguenot Zamariel/de la Roche-Chandieu claimed infected the poet, to reveal the physical and moral degradation of the Huguenot preacher and his colleagues, and by extension, their theology. He offers an open scrutiny—a public confession—of his life, both virtues and vices, as if to refute the Calvinist perception that Catholics are unwilling to confess in public: "Tu te plains d'autre-part que ma vie est lascive, / . . . Or je veux que ma vie en escrit apparaisse" ("Response aux injures," II: 606, v. 18, v. 22) [You complain too that my life is wanton, / . . . But I want my life to appear in writing].[24] The poet proceeds to highlight his daily routine: prayers, study, writing, Mass, walks in nature, and, until suppressed in 1573, his enjoyment of the company of women, a detail that, as Gustave Cohen notes, assures the sincerity and completeness of his confession (606, n. 18). In contrast to his own lifestyle, with its virtues and vices, he blames the hypocrisy that characterizes the habits of his accuser—turning a profit from the Scriptures, flattering young nuns with seductive words, taking advantage of lowly monks, and appropriating what belongs to God:

> Tu sçais de l'Evangile engraisser tes mains,
> Tu sçais bien enjoller quelques jeunes nonnains,
> Tu sçais bien desfroquer la simplesse d'un moine,
> Et convertir au tien de Dieu le patrimoine;
> ("Response aux injures," II: 616, vv. 38–41)

Ronsard takes issue with the presumption ("cuider") and the overriding confidence that the Calvinists place in human reasoning, a trait that leads them to believe they alone are the chosen people: "Tu as en Paradis le tiers et les deux pars / Tu en es fils aisné, nous en sommes bastars" (II: 616, vv. 39–40). I have come full circle from the accusations of the early evangelical humanists such as Briçonnet, Rabelais, and Marguerite de Navarre, who blamed the presumption ("cuider") of the Catholic theologians. Frank Lestringat remarks on how Ronsard reproaches the Calvinist reliance on "raison naturelle" over " les lumières de la foi" in refusing both transubstantiation and the Lutheran notion of ubiquity—where Christ is present both at the Mass and seated in heaven on the right hand of God (*Une sainte horreur,* 180).

As I shall show later with Montaigne and Agrippa d'Aubigné, Ronsard looks to the health of France, the unity of the people, the stability of the law, the harmony that comes from obedience to a single monarch and a unified faith.[25] He denounces Calvinism for untying the cord that binds the people in peace: "Or c'est là, predicant, l'Evangile et le fruict / Que ta nouvelle secte en la France a produit, / Rompant toute amitié et desnoüant la corde / Qui fortement serroit les peuples en concorde" ("Response aux injures," II: 608, vv. 30–33). He evokes the recent peace organized by the queen mother, the Paix d'Amboise of 1563, and his hope that it will restore France's strength and vigor as a soft rain restores a flower wilted by the same hot sun that renders humankind feverish and thirsty:

> Mais la paix que la Royne heureusement a faite,
> L'a remise en vigueur et sa force a refaite,
> Comme une douce pluye en sa vertu remet
> La fleur espanouye à qui jà le sommet
> Pendoit flestry du chaud, quand le Soleil ameine
> Les fievres et la soif à nostre race humaine.
> ("Response aux injures," II: 602, vv. 42–43, 603, vv. 1–4)

In replying to his accuser, the poet strengthens his argument by stating that while Zamariel believes only in his own personal view, Ronsard founds his belief on the more solid, common, Catholic union: "Car tu crois seulement en ton opinion / Moy en la catholique et publique union" (II: 609, vv. 15–16). His rhetoric is grounded in the opposition between private and public, singular and common, sedition and obedience. France's law is founded in and strengthened by the connection between religion and monarch. Discord arises from advancing the personal over the common good.

> Tu m'estimes meschant, et meschant je t'estime,
> Je retourne sur toy le mesme faict du crime;
> Tu penses que c'est moy, je pense que c'est toy;
> Et qui fait ce discord? nostre diverse foy.
> (II: 609, vv. 9–12)

> You judge me evil and evil I judge you,
> I put on you the same crime,
> You think it is I and I think it is you;
> And what causes this discord? Our differing beliefs.

The disagreement and mistrust that exists between these two thinkers and writers is a microcosm of the larger discord that tears France apart. At one time, to be French was to espouse a common faith, a common interpretation of the Gospels. Diversity of belief for Ronsard introduces an imbalance in the system of justice.

The focus of this book—syphilis as a metaphor for religious controversy—demands a different context from that which Ullrich Langer brought to his insightful study of Ronsard's "Response aux injures et calomnies": the public and private activities of the courtier.[26] Here I note the clever way in which Ronsard, while setting his vigor against Zamariel's pallor, promotes, along with the pleasure the poet takes in courtly activities, his humility in obedience both to "l'Eternel, le pere de tout bien" and to the "loix de mon Prince" (II: 606). He contrasts his restraint and devotion to his two princes—one eternal, the other temporal—with the excess of Huguenot deceit, heresy, and cruelty. His task is to respond to and blame his accusers.[27]

> Blasmant les predicans qui seuls avoyent presché
> Que par le fer mutin le peuple fust tranché,
> Blasmant les assassins, les volleurs et l'outrage
> Des hommes reformez, cruels en brigandage...
> (II: 619, vv. 5–8)

> Casting blame on the preachers who only preached
> That by the mutinous sword the people were felled,
> Casting blame on the assassins, the thiefs, and the abuse
> Of the men of the Reform, cruel in pillaging...

The accusation of syphilis, disseminated by the Huguenots, becomes a pretext for Ronsard to lash out at what he perceives to be the errors of the theologians of Geneva.

Infection and epidemic had seized the imagination of French intellectuals—whether on the side of the Catholics or the Protestants. As Jeff Persels has pointed out, "Given that this current age so often has recourse to metaphors of illness . . . we should not be . . . surprised to find earlier ages equally devoted to the figurative potential of mortal infirmity" (Persels, 1089). Narratives coming back from the New World of the "paillardise" and "luxure" of the indigenous populations became intertwined with the hyperbolic language used by the Protestants or Catholics in accusing their enemies of excesses, whether of a sexual or gastronomic nature. Spiritual and carnal corruption had rendered the kingdom sick. At a much later date following the death of Henri IV, Agrippa d'Aubigné would say as religious strife resumed: "Le royaume est malade par la subversion de toutes choses." [The kingdom is sickened by the subversion of all things].[28] Participants in the Wars of Religion appropriated the vocabulary from the syphilis pandemic to describe the physical and spiritual malaise that characterized the conflict. It is perhaps an instance of early recognition, to use Thevet's words, of "un mal commun à tout le monde" [a worldwide disease] (Thevet, 211). From the perspective of those chronicling the disease either in the Old World or the New, it was a global sickness brought on by the failure of people to heed a common set of moral values. It was also a recognition that, with the discovery of the *Terres Neufves*, the age of common values had passed.

4

Wild Appetites/Appétit[s] Desordonné[s][1]
Cannibalism, Siege, and the Sins of the Old World in Jean de Léry

> Mais j'ai l'impression d'une connivance, d'un parallélisme entre l'existence de Léry et la mienne.
> —*Entretien avec Claude Lévi-Strauss*[2]

To UNDERSTAND how cannibalism, and by association, syphilis, took such a strong hold on the imagination and language of Catholics and Protestants alike during the French Wars of Religion, it is necessary to follow the thoughts and writing of the man whose writings Claude Lévi-Strauss said inspired his own explorations, the early ethnographer and Protestant pastor Jean de Léry. While Lévi-Strauss encourages the reading of Léry as "une grande oeuvre littéraire," leaving ethnography to the ethnographers, he notes several qualities that seem to establish Léry's ethnographic perceptions: he gives himself to the revelations of the land he is exploring ("Il y a eu chez lui une sorte de révélation du terrain"); he exhibits astonishment at unfamiliar things ("Il a su s'emerveiller des choses inouïes"); and he has an eye and a capacity to see and to record accurately ("le regard de Léry . . . sa capacité de voir"). This is in contrast to his ideological rival, Franciscan cosmographer Thevet, who often relied on information gathered by others without passing it through the filter of his own experiential observations: "Du coup, la différence entre les deux hommes, entre les deux visions qu'ils proposent, vient de l'oeil de Léry: à l'instar de l'éthnologue, il a fait passer ses expérience avant les informations de seconde main qu'il recueillait" ("Entretien," 8–9) [As a result, the difference between the two men, between the two visions that they propose, comes from Léry's eye: in the manner of the ethnologist, his own experiences take precedence over the second hand information he gathers]. As Lévi-Strauss and others point out, Thevet's objective was boastful self-aggrandizement ("vantardises"), Léry's to observe and appreciate ("Entretien," 9).

Pinpointing the evolution of Léry's thoughts on cannibalism is rendered somewhat problematic by the fact that his *Histoire memorable du Siège de Sancerre,* published in 1574, predates his *Histoire d'un voyage faict en la terre du Brésil,* published first in 1578. He notes in his *préface* to the latter work that he had in fact redacted a first version in 1563, an expansion of his notes written "d'ancre de Brésil, et en l'Amerique mesme" [with brazilwood ink, and in America itself], and then wrote a second version to replace the first, which had been confiscated at the gates of Lyon.³ This second version was also lost in the haste with which he left to take refuge in Sancerre to escape religious persecution as a Protestant. It was only in 1576 that he was able to rework the text when the second version was returned to him through the efforts of a prominent lord ("un notable seigneur"; *Histoire d'un voyage,* 61–62).

Montaigne follows Léry in observing that the indigenous people of Brazil, the Tupinamba, are motivated not by hunger but by ritual in consuming the body pieces of their enemies: "Ce n'est pas, comme on pense, pour s'en nourrir, ainsi que faisoient anciennement les Scythes: c'est pour representer une extreme vengeance" [This is not, as people think, for nourishment, as of old the Scythians used to do; it is to betoken an extreme revenge].⁴ Having described the cooking of the flesh of the enemy prisoner on the grill or *boucan,* Léry states that the Tupinamba ate not for nourishment ("ayans esgard à la nourriture"), even though they all attested to the meat being "good and delicate" ("merveilleusement bonne et delicate"), but for reasons of vengeance against the enemy people ("plus par vengeance"; *Histoire d'un voyage,* 365–66/127). The Tupinamba sought to make an example "to strike fear and terror into the hearts of the livings" ("ils donnent par ce moyen crainte et espouvantement aux vivans"; 366/127). Other evidence of this extreme vengeance is seen in rubbing the "bodies, arms, thighs, and legs" of the Tupinamba children "with the blood of the enemies" to inspire the same vengeance in the children ("frottent le corps, bras, cuisses et jambes du sang de leurs ennemis"; 362/126) and in killing the offspring of the women who had served as sexual companions to the prisoners held captive since they came from enemy seed ("tels enfans sont provenus de la semence de leurs ennemis"; 369/128).

Léry captures the ritual value of the process—both in describing the pride of the captive ready to die valiantly, jumping and drinking as part of the dances surrounding the symbolic ceremony ("sautant et buvant il sera des plus joyeux"; *Histoire d'un voyage,* 355/122). As Montaigne would do in reworking the accounts of the New World chroniclers, Léry assesses the "cruauté des sauvages" in the light of similar cruelties in the Old World: "our big usurers" "sucking the blood and marrow and eating everyone alive—widows, orphans, and other poor people" ("nos gros usuriers" "sucçans le sang et la moëlle, et par consequent mangeans tous en vie, tand de vefves, orphelins et autre pauvres personnes"; *Histoire d'un voyage,* 375/132). Similarly, he points to the savage persecution of Huguenots in Lyon and Auxerre. He depicts images of livers, hearts, and other body parts cut into pieces and consumed, only because these people professed to belonging to the "Religion reformée" (376/132).[5] Géralde Nakam invokes the rationalism, as strong in Léry as it is in Montaigne, that refuses to take refuge in supernatural explanations when it is human aggression that is at fault (Léry, *Histoire mémorable du Siège de Sancerre,* 103). Nakam points out that Léry and Montaigne look to the "victimes d'agression" (*Au lendemain de la Saint-Barthélemy,* 84) and plead their cause. This rationalism allows Léry to understand that the nudity of the Tupinamba women is no less damaging than the elaborate fashion accessories of the French women, including "paint, wigs, curled hair, ruffs, farthinggales" ("fards, fausses perruques, cheveux tortillez, grands collets fraisez, vertugales"; *Histoire d'un voyage,* 234/67).[6] What some might see as rationalism, Levi-Strauss calls Léry's eye—his power of observation, a tool that allows him to appreciate the natural beauty of the nude Tupinamba women over the artificial and excessive grooming habits of European women.

The notations of sadness are introduced by Léry, motivated as he is by his European sensitivities to preparing human flesh for consumption: "Pour la fin de ceste tant estrange tragedie," "chose horrible à ouir, et encor plus à voir" (369/128) [To conclude this strange tragedy, (a) horrible thing to hear and what follows is even worse to see]. He anticipates the reader's shock but does not let it interfere with his attempts to capture the tone of the Tupinamban ceremonies. As Claude Lévi-Strauss says in the above referenced interview, "Le secret, c'est qu'il s'est mis dans la peau des Indiens" ("Entretien," *Histoire d'un voyage,* 11).

Fright and horror comes from the French side in witnessing the act of cannibalism; joy and courage emerges from the indigenous Brazilians. Léry makes it very clear that there is a middle ground—a murky place where the interpreters who have lived among the Brazilians long enough to pick up their language have also begun to appropriate their practices, but outside of the ritualistic system of the Tupinamba. Again, this middle ground is expressed in religious terms—atheism. Léry and his fellow Reformed Christians are careful not to partake of the grilled human flesh of the enemies of the Tupinamba. This refusal runs against the natural generosity of the Brazilians to feed their allies and to distribute the body pieces to everyone ("quelque grand qu'en soit le nombre chacun, s'il est possible, avant que sortir de là en aura son morceau" [*Histoire d'un voyage*, 365/127] [However many of them there are, each of them will, if possible, have his morsel]). To refuse was to be suspected of being disloyal ("il leur sembloit par cela que nous ne fussions pas assez loyaux" [370/128] [it seemed to them that we were not showing proper loyalty]). The interpreters ("truchemens") from Normandy showed no such reticence and boasted of have killed and eaten prisoners ("se vantoyent d'avoir tué et mangé des prisonniers"; 370/128). The disapproving pastor Léry attributes the cause to their living "une vie d'Atheistes," forgetting their own Christian rituals during the eight or nine years of their stay, which in turn leads them to lecherous living with the Tupinamba women and girls ("ne se polluant pas seulement en toutes sortes de paillardises et vilenies parmi les femmes et les filles"; 370/128). One of the Normans is involved with a boy three years old. Cannibalism within its cultural context is one thing, but by being practiced by those who come from another culture and by those who have abandoned their faith, it surpasses, through this disrespectful and detached imitation, the inhumanity of the indigenous practice ("surpassans les sauvages en inhumanité"; 370/128).

Villegagnon, commanding the French in Brazil, had expressly prohibited every Christian ("nul ayant titre de Chrestien") from sleeping with the Tupinamba women. But the Norman interpreters were hard to control, as Léry reports in chapter 6, where Villegagnon orders that a Norman "truchement" be hung rather than tortured "pour avoir paillardé" with a Tupinamba woman (*Histoire d'un voyage*, 181/43). Léry uncharacteristically praises Villegagnon for having forbidden such liaisons, although he does mention that others—probably Protestant—accused the leader of "having defiled himself" with the indigenous women ("que

quand il estoit en l'Amerique il se polluoit avec les femmes sauvages";
181/43), a fact of which Léry says he had no knowledge.[7] Villegagnon
had reason beyond the fact that these women were not Christian to forbid his men from consorting with them. In chapter 19, Léry, like Thevet, describes the incurable illness that they call *Pians,* "laquelle combien qu'ordinairement elle se prenne et provienne de paillardise, j'ay neantmoins veu avoir à des jeunes enfans qui en estoyent aussi couverts" (*Histoire d'un voyage,* 469).[8] The detailed description of "postules plus larges que le pouce, lesquelles s'espandent par tout le corps et jusques au visage" makes it clear that it is the same pox from which "les verolez et chancreux" [syphilitics and poxy ones] suffer in Europe ("de par deçà").

Léry's description conforms to the observations of two of his medical contemporaries: Ambroise Paré and Jean Fernel. Paré refers to the "quelque ulcere dans les parties honteuses . . . & quelquesfois tout le corps" [sores in the private parts . . . and sometimes over the whole body.][9] Fernel uses the term "postules" and speaks of them as being "sans nombre, rugueuses, saillantes, comparable pour la forme et la grandeur à des glands de chêne" [pustules; countless, rough, protruding, comparable in form and size to acorns].[10] Léry, like the learned physicians, knew that the pox endangered not only the men and women who engaged in sexual relationships but also nursing children. In depicting the lax morals and adaptability of the Norman interpreters to Tupi customs, Léry connects their appropriation or perverse imitation of cannibalism with their wanton relationships with the Tupinamba women, in spite of Villegagnon's interdiction. Had the Norman "truchemens" remained true to their culture—to the teachings of Christ and their French customs—they would not have engaged in cannibalism, nor in fact contracted the pox. The pollution comes from the unnatural act of eating one's own species—human flesh—along with committing wanton "paillardise."[11] As Nakam says of his *Histoire mémorable,* "Léry refuse d'être écrivain: à aucun moment il ne veut ni ne peut séparer en lui le chroniqueur du moraliste" (82) [Léry refuses to be a writer; at no time does he wish to nor can he separate the chronicler from the moralist in him].

Adverse circumstances such as the absence of French women or familiar food in Brazil or the scarcity of food imposed by the Catholics besieging Sancerre are no excuse for lapsed morals or for violating basic moral principles. Without boasting, Léry makes a point that, with the exception of the "truchemens," the Reformed Christians and the men of Villegagnon followed the interdictions for avoiding both sexual liaisons with the

Tupi women and the consumption of human flesh. As to the first instance, he asserts that "Neantmoins, comme ceste loy avoit doublement son fondement sur la parole de Dieu, aussi fut-elle si bien observée, que non seulement pas un seul des gens de Villegagon ny de nostre compagnie ne la transgressa" (*Histoire d'un voyage*, 181/43) [Nevertheless, as this law also had its foundation in the word of God, so was it so well-observed that not only did none of Villegagnon's men nor [members] of our group violate it]. Léry is scrupulous in mentioning that he and his men avoided consuming human flesh. He describes his horror at being awakened and handed a foot of a prisoner cooked over the grill ("un pied d'icelluy cuict et boucané"; 452). The fright exhibited by "Big Oyster" (Lery-oussou, the Tupi version of Léry's name) made plain his refusal of the proffered morsel. In the *Histoire mémorable du siège de Sancerre*, published four years prior to the *Histoire d'un voyage*, he notes his own horror when surprising the Potard family getting ready to eat their daughter's "deux cuisses, jambes et pieds dans une chaudiere" (291) [two thighs, legs, and feet in a pot]. Léry paints his fright in a manner that makes clear the moral implications of this act of cannibalism: "Je fus si effroyé et esperdu que toutes mes entrailles en furent esmeues" (291). Another time, "un quidam pressé de faim me demanda à Sancerre, s'il ne feroit point mal, et n'offenseroit Dieu de manger en ceste extreme necessité de la fesse d'un homme qui avoit esté tué, laquelle luy sembloit si belle" (*Histoire mémorable du siège de Sancerre*, 295) [a certain fellow desperate with hunger asked me if it wouldn't cause any harm nor offend God if he ate in this extreme necessity the buttocks of a man who had been killed and seemed so appealing to him]. Finding the proposition odious, Léry leaves it to the boy's scruples and conscience to interpret the proper response by telling him that even animals—wolves, for example—don't eat their own kind ("je luy alleguay les bestes pour exemple, et les loups qu'on dit qui ne se mangent l'un l'autre"; 296). On the subject of cannibalism, Léry is seen as someone who has witnessed it but who is also a strong moral arbiter in his opposition to seeing it practiced by Christians. The link is clear between the proffered foot, grilled to perfection in Brazil, and the simmering body parts chez Potard or the dismembered buttocks in Sancerre.

It is not the sensationalism that brings Léry, or Montaigne, for that matter, back to the shocking imagery of cannibalism. It is the compelling moral argument that the image provides. For Léry, the person with gives himself or herself to cannibalism, even in the face of near-starvation, gives up French cultural heritage: millennia of the Judeo-Christian teachings. The Norman "truchemens" in Brazil gave themselves both to "paillardise" and cannibalism. While the Potard family could have chosen to get along on herb soup and boiled belts in the manner of the other Christians—Reformed and other—they let themselves yield to their "appetit desordonné." As was seen with the Norman "truchemens," their barbarity is all the more savage and inhumane because there is no compelling cultural context. The Tupinamba do not eat their own relatives; they avenge the aggression of their enemies through the act of cannibalism. In speaking about Monsieur and Madame Potard and the old woman, Léry states:

> Brief que non seulement la famine, mais aussi un appetit desordonné leur avoit faict commettre ceste cruauté barbare et plus que bestiale: le mary et la femme estans aussi de long temps mal renommez, tenus pour yvrognes, gourmands, et mesmes cruels envers leurs enfans.

> Briefly not only famine, but also a uncontrolled appetite made them commit this savage and beyond bestial cruelty, since the husband and wife had long enjoyed a bad reputation, considered drunks, gluttons, and even cruel towards their children. (*Histoire memorable*, 292)

There is a middle ground represented by the Norman interpreters—"menans une vie d'Atheistes" (*Histoire d'un voyage*, 370). Like the Norman interpreters in Brazil, the Potard polluted themselves with every vice outlined in the laws of Moses. In contrast, the response of the Protestant inhabitants of Sancerre to the cruel starvation caused by the siege and by the Catholics is exemplary:

> Toutesfois au milieu de ceste grande destresse et calamité, on en voyoit de merveilleusement constans, et faisans ces exclamations, "Helas Seigneur delivre nous de ces fleaux, et verges de famine et de guerre dont tu nous bas et chaties justement à cause de nos pechez. Aye pitié de ton pauvre peuple, et au milieu de ton ire souvienne-toy de ta misericorde." (*Histoire mémorable*, 298)

> Still in the middle of this great distress and calamity, wonderfully constant people were seen making these entreaties: "Alas Lord deliver us from these blights and rods of famine and war with which you beat us and punish us justly for our sins. Have pity on your poor people and in the midst of your rage remember your mercy."

The steadfast Huguenot invocations to the Lord both underscore original sin and stress the message of God's unconditional mercy, detached as it is from any notion of good works. Before Montaigne, Léry appropriates the literal and metaphorical dimensions of cannibalism to reflect the religious tensions present in France at the time of the wars of religion.

To better understand how Léry came to engage the image of cannibalism in the religious and civil violence in France, it is necessary to study just how comments about cannibalism in the *Histoire mémorable du siège de Sancerre* both recall to his readers his role as a missionary and an observer to the indigenous peoples of Brazil and prepare us for his own chronicles of his stay there. We may remain skeptical when he tells us at its publication in 1578 that he had not originally intended to publish his own account but felt compelled to in order to counter the lies found in Thevet's work. Franciscan by training, cosmographer of the king, and chaplain to Catherine de Medici, Thevet represents those who persecute the Protestants. Léry goes on to say that he might have let the lies and errors contained in the first edition of Thevet's *Singularitez de la France Antarctique* (1557) pass unanswered if he had not encountered further lies condemning the actions of the Reformed pastors in Thevet's reworking of the early chronicles in the *Cosmographie universelle* (1575).[12]

Léry is somewhat singular in creating a dialogue between his *Histoire mémorable du siège de Sancerre* and the *Histoire d'un voyage faict en la terre du Brésil,* published four years later, as I have noted. Was he afraid that people would have forgotten his valiant and perilous efforts to bring the Tupinamba into the Christian fold? Or did he wish to establish himself as the French expert on Tupi mores, including cannibalism? At the very least, his cross-references are tied to his earnest efforts to promote his Huguenot faith. In any event, there is a continual going back and forth between what Léry was witnessing in Sancerre and what he had witnessed in Brazil, and thus for the post-1578 reader, a strong link between the two works.

It is not surprising that Léry sought to, in Géralde Nakam's words, "isoler le phénomène de la faim" (*Au lendemain de la Saint-Barthélemy,* 100) [isolate the phenomenon of hunger] in all its manifestations through linking it with his previous experience of extreme starvation on board the ship returning from Brazil. His status as a missionary and an ethnographer of the New World would bring him both notice and notoriety from Catholic royal forces besieging Sancerre. But Léry established in his own voice his expertise on hunger—his reliability as a witness to the suffering of the besieged in Sancerre:

Au retour d'un Voyage que je feis en la terre du Bresil dite Amerique, en l'an 1558, ayans demeurez et branslez cinq mois sur mer sans mettre pied à terre, et durant la famine que nous eusmes d'un mois, nos fusmes contraincts de manger des rondaches de cuir sec, faites de la peau d'un animal gros comme un taureau d'un an que les Sauvages appelent Tapiroussou, mais nous les mettions seulement rostir sur les charbons par petits morceaus: et ne peusmes trouver l'invention de les amollir comme nous avons faict les peaux seiches à Sancerre. (*Histoire mémorable du siège de Sancerre*, 284)

On the return from a voyage that I made to the land of Brazil, called America, in the year 1558, having remained rocking five months on the sea without setting foot on land and during the month's famine that we endured, we were forced to eat dried leather shields made of the skin of an animal as big as a bull that the Savages call *Tapiroussou;* but we only roasted it on small pieces of coal and didn't manage to soften them as we did the dried skins in Sancerre.

I take the time to cite the entire passage because, in its precision as to the date and destination, Léry connects the two experiences—Brazil and Sancerre, and reminds his readers that he brings the experience of chronicler/ethnographer/missionary to Sancerre. At the same time, he refuses to credit himself with showing the besieged people how to make it through the famine. In fact, the leader of the besiegers would later try to pin on Léry the crime of prolonging the resistance through the tricks he had learned in the New World. This Léry, as shall be seen, patently denies and instead here, as he will do later in the account, he credits the "invention," the inventive spirit of the people of Sancerre and the refugees from persecution in Catholic France. The long aside is key to setting the "phenomenon of hunger" in place and permits him to be somewhat less detailed when referencing his Brazilian trip farther along in the account.

He contrasts the adult experiences of the missionary explorers and trained soldiers who went to the New World with the youthful inventiveness of the boys of Sancerre, who turned their leather belts into nourishment: "Les enfants aussi qui avoyent des ceinctures de cuir les mettoyent sur les charbons, et s'en desjunoyent comme d'un boyau de tripes" (*Histoire mémorable du siège de Sancerre,* 287) [The children, too who had leather belts set them on the coals and dined on them as if they were tripe guts]. Whether Léry knew that this heartrending image of the youths sacrificing their belts for food would become iconic in the Reformed pamphlets and poetry of the time—a symbol of the sacrifice, courage, faith, and invention of the besieged—one can only guess. There is also the playful aspect of tripe, for those readers who recalled Rabelais's joyful account of Gargamelle's labor brought on from having eaten too much tripe: "par trop avoir mangé des trippes." This of course produces the happy birth of Gargantua—another inventive youth (*Gargantua*, 56).

Another link between the *Histoire mémorable de Sancerre* and the *Histoire d'un voyage faict en la terre de Brésil* occurs in a culminating spot of the narrative of hunger—the account of the single act of cannibalism carried out during the siege, when the Potard family and the old woman ate the body pieces of their baby girl. Just following the passage quoted above, in which Léry talks about his fright and the upsetting effect on his "entrailles," he again references his travels to Brazil: "Car combien que j'aye demeuré dix mois entre les Sauvages Ameriquains en la terre du Bresil, leur ayant veu souvent manger de la chair humaine, (d'autant qu'ils mangent les prisonniers qu'ils prennent en guerre) si n'en ay-je jamais eu telle terreur que j'eus frayeur de voir ce piteux spectacle, lequel n'avoit encores (comme je croy) jamais esté veu en ville assiegée en nostre France" (*Histoire mémorable du siège de Sancerre*, 291) [Since even though I have spent ten months among the American Savages in the land of Brazil, having seen them often eat human flesh (in as much as they eat the prisoners that they capture in war), so I have never felt such terror as the fright I felt in seeing this pitiful spectacle, which, as I believe, has never before been seen in France in a city under siege]. Léry reminds his readers that cannibalism is a part of the ritual of war in Brazil and that the prisoners are not family members but enemies. The practice of eating the flesh of one's species, however much against both human nature and even animal nature, is anchored in ritual vengeance. The Potard parents—an exception even in France—exceeded the savagery of the inhabitants of the New World in eating their own child for nourishment, in violation of all religious commandments. As if to highlight "ce crime prodigieux barbare et inhumain" [the prodigal, savage and inhuman crime] against God's Law ("sa Loy"), Léry describes the crime in great detail from his perspective, as one might describe a feast—including the vinegar, spices, and salt simmering in the pot with the body parts:

> *Ayant veu* l'os et le test de la teste de ceste pauvre fille, curé, et rongé, et les oreilles mangées, *ayant veu aussi* la langue cuite, espesse d'un doigt,

qu'ils estoyent prests à manger, quand ils furent surpris: les deux cuisses, jambes et pieds dans une chaudiere avec vinaigre, espices et sel, prests à cuire et mettre sur le feu. (*Histoire mémorable du siège de Sancerre*, 291)

Having seen the scalp of the head of this poor girl, cured and gnawed and the ears eaten, *having seen as well* the cooked tongue, thick as a finger, that they were ready to eat when they were surprised: the two thighs, legs and feet in a pot with vinegar, spices and salt, ready to cook and put on the fire.

The pastor brings the careful eye of the ethnographer to witness what will become a major piece of the iconographic story of the Catholic persecution of the Protestants. He portrays his fright and revulsion on seeing the broken and open chest of the tiny girl ("La poitrine fendue et ouverte"; 291). The image evokes how one might break open a chicken breast to lay on the fire. Léry's perspective is just one person's testimony to the wild appetite ("appetit desordonné"; 292) of the Potard parents and the old lady. Yet the skilled and engaged narrator describes it for all to witness.

Léry continues to link his experiences with cannibalism in Brazil to his witnessing of famine in Sancerre through his comments about the old lady Philippes de la Feüille. He tells us that, according to the Potard husband, he was led on ("incité") to commit the cannibalism by Philippes—an explanation that rings true to Léry, since in Brazil, the old Tupinamba women ate with greater appetite and relish the flesh of the enemy captives than the men and younger women and children: "J'ay observé estant avec les Sauvages Ameriquains, que les vieilles femmes de ces pays là sont beaucoup plus friandes, appetent et souhaittent plus de manger de la chair humaines que les hommes, ny que les jeunes femmes et enfans" (*Histoire mémorable du siège de Sancerre, 295*). When Léry returned to redact the stories of his travels to Brazil, he would use the same word to describe the enthusiasm with which the old women gave themselves to consuming human flesh—"friandes": "hormis ce que j'ay dit particulierement des vieilles femmes qui en sont si friandes" (*Histoire d'un voyage*, 366/126) [who (as I have said) have an amazing appetite for human flesh]. Recycling imagery at key dramatic moments of an account is one way of linking the two *Histoires*.

The attribution of appetite to cannibalism is problematic, since Léry had said that the Tupinamba ate not for nourishment but to show vengeance to their enemies. Frank Lestringant observes that Léry creates an exception to the symbolic, ritualistic meaning of cannibalism in speaking of the old women's appetite for human flesh (366, n. 1). The attribution blurs an otherwise clean line between the indigenous Brazilians, who ate generally within the symbolic ritual of vengeance, and the Potard family and the old woman Philippes, who ate and disobeyed God's Law out of human weakness and gluttony. They alone of all the god-fearing Christians in Sancerre disrespected thousands of years of prohibition of consuming the flesh of one's own kind. What further troubles the citizens "de l'ordre de l'Eglise reformée" was that the Potards had taken advantage of the charitable gift of herb soup and wine like many other hungry villagers and so had no reason to commit this "acte prodigieux": "Ils avoyent eu l'aumosne d'un potage d'herbes, et du vin competemment . . . et veu la necessité où chascun estoit reduict, cela estoit suffisant pour passer ceste journée: brief que non seulement la famine, mais aussi un appetit desordonné leur avoit faict commettre ceste cruauté barbare et plusque bestiale" (292). In the narration of the act of cannibalism committed by the Potard family, it turns out that not only is M. Potard guilty of theft and murder, but he and Mme. Potard may have committed bigamy, for in not wanting to wait to marry before news of her former husband Sacré's death, as the Consistory of the Reformed Church required, they were married by the Catholic Church ("ils s'allerent espouser à la papauté"; 292). So in fact, the lapse in humane behavior—this bestial act of cannibalism—was performed by Catholics. As Léry had attributed the cannibalism of the Norman interpreters to their atheism, here he explains the Potards' wild appetite as a function of their return to the papacy. In contrast to the profligacy of the *famille,* Potard stand the prayers of the besieged Huguenots, who entreat the Lord to help them bear his punishment and to receive his mercy.[13]

Inserted in the narrative but not emphasized by Léry was the fact that he enjoyed both renown and notoriety among the leaders who besieged Sancerre because of his travels to Brazil. He was pulled aside and questioned—some might say given preferential treatment—during the conclusion of the siege. As the siege was ending, Claude de La Châtre, the leader, took the pastor aside and accused him of having incited the people of Sancerre to hold out ("faict opiniastrer ceux de Sancerre"). La Châtre believed Léry had shown them how to eat leathers and skins, as he had done crossing the ocean on the route back from Brazil: "Leur ayant enseigné la façon de manger les cuirs et peaux, ainsi que j'avois autrefois fait sur mer, au retour de la terre de Bresil" (*Histoire mémorable du siège de Sancerre,* 327). Now it is known from Léry's own account that he had shared his expertise—a fact detailed above—but he continued to maintain that the ingenuity of the people of Sancerre far surpassed his knowledge: "Je luy fis response que sans me vouloir excuser, que je n'eusse faict tout ce que j'avois peu et deu dans Sancerre, je n'avois pas trouvé cette invention, et n'y avoit eu autre industrie pour manger les peaux et autres choses encores plus estranges, dont nous avions vescu, depuis quelque temps, que la necessité maistresse des arts" (327). Necessity is indeed the mother of invention—it was animal skins or starvation. Léry turns the rebuke into a glimpse of the valor of the people as they resisted the Catholic forces.

It is La Châtre's response that gives rise to Léry's account of the siege. La Châtre says that he bears Léry no ill will but would like to have an account of the methods by which the people withstood the siege. Léry takes advantage of the interview to strongly justify the position of the Protestants—"ceux de la Religion." He bids La Châtre to consider the principal—the justice and equity of the Huguenot cause ("la justice et equité de nostre cause"). The refugee Huguenots such as himself had never misbehaved or transgressed the royal edict ("sans avoir mesfaict, ny transgressé l'Edict du Roy"). Their only choice after the cruel treatment was to take refuge in Sancerre, where they took up no arms for six weeks and then only in self-defense (*Histoire mémorable du siège de Sancerre*, 328). For La Châtre, the blame for starvation lies with the obstinacy of the besieged in holding out for so long ("nous ne nous pouvions excuser de ce que nous avions faict, ayans tenu si long temps sans vouloir rendre la place"; 328). To the point that peace could have been achieved earlier, when Monsieur de Saint Pierre spoke to Léry, Léry remains firm in his defense of the actions of the Huguenots—how could they trust the man's word when all they had heard from the Catholic cause was to "exterminer ceux de la Religion"? (329). That Léry was considered an extraordinary person by the besiegers is clear, but the pastor did not take advantage of his position. Instead he gave a strong accounting to justify the actions and right of the Huguenots to exercise their freedom of conscience in a world intent on destroying them and their faith.[14] He was witness to the strength of their belief in their "cause."

The rigor of La Châtre's accusation, in spite of his remark that he will not hold a grudge against Léry, stands in contrast to the good humor of the maître du camp Sarrieu. Sarrieu and his men invite Léry among other Huguenot leaders to dine. They are well treated, and Sarrieu has the good grace to laugh and appreciate Léry's wit when he comments that the Huguenots consider this event one of God's marvels: those who had come hoping to kill and slit the throats of the Huguenots were now like fathers taking care to restore them after the hard and bitter famine they had suffered: "que nous voyons en cela les merveilles de Dieu, qui avoit tellement besongné, que ceux qui estoyent venus en esperance de nous tuer et esgorger, nous estoyent comme peres nourrissiers, apres une dure et aspre famine que nous avions soufferte" (*Histoire mémorable du siège de Sancerre*, 335). In Sarrieu and Léry can be seen the sense of humor that comes with modesty—the opposite of that overwhelming certitude and presumption ("le cuyder") so evident in La Châtre. Léry attributes the survival of the people to the justice of the cause and to God's grace.[15] Sarrieu has the good sense to recognize the humility of his Huguenot counterparts and, in good humor, admit that he and his men were not as bad as they had been made out to be ("n'estoyent si mauvais qu'on les faisoit"; 335). Léry becomes a witness to the members of the enemy camp, and by extension to all his readers, of the power of the divine spirit that ran through the siege and gave the besieged the strength to persevere against all odds.

Andrea Frisch describes the influence of Calvin's theory of the power of witness by the Holy Spirit during the Eucharist, which allows the communicant to feel the symbolic presence of the Lord in the host and the wine (Frisch, 90). This is not the literal presence of the body and blood, as the Catholic ideology holds. Frisch shows how Calvin's concept of witness carries into Léry's ethnography: "Léry's appropriation of Calvin's 'spiritual' mode of testimony constitutes the most remarkable ethnographic achievement of the *Histoire d'un voyage faict en la terre de Brésil*" (Frisch, 90). One manner of witnessing is carried out through self-citation, and while Frisch shows how this works in the Brazil narrative, she does not extend it to the narrative of the siege of Sancerre. I will take her notion of "self-citation," expand it to include the account of the siege of Sancerre, and show how in the context of Sancerre, Léry's witnessing evokes the divine spirit that allows the Huguenots to survive. The play of one *Histoire* against the other enhances the impact of both works.

The above examples from the *Histoire mémorable du siège de Sancerre*, referencing Léry's journey and experiences in Brazil and also citing members of the enemy camp in the siege referencing Léry's experiences in Brazil, amount to what Frisch refers to as "self-citation." Nakam's allusion to the legendary status that had arisen around the personality of Léry precisely because of his travels to Brazil helps to clarify why Léry would take up the practice of self-citation. If the great captains of Catholic royal history in France invoked his experience and sought his advice, then the uniqueness of his account and opinion is evident. As Frisch states, "Léry's citations of his own text function as authoritative witnesses to the reliability of his report" (Frisch, 95). As I have mentioned earlier, the continual citing of a not-yet-written experience—at least in its definitive and published form—to enhance the authority of the Sancerre text as it unfolds simulates the inspiration that breathes through the author as he endeavors to recount the struggles of his people to survive. La Châtre's request for the account of the struggle reinforces the notion that this is not the particular experience of an individual or a group, but an experience that can serve to instruct and inspire others.[16] It takes on, as many of the episodes in Montaigne's *Essais* do, an "atemporal quality," a term used by Frisch.

Something that gives this "atemporal quality" is the effort to develop a psychology of famine at the end of the *Histoire d'un voyage faict en la terre du Brésil*. In the *Histoire mémorable du siège de Sancerre,* in contrast, Léry retains his role of witness to the persecution of the Huguenots without probing what goes on in the minds of human beings when faced by extreme hunger. Perhaps the distance from events, both in Brazil and in Sancerre, and the further persecution of "ceux de la religion" leads him to try to understand the phenomenon of cannibalism in these extreme events through the words of the Old Testament. To aid his thought process, he again gives himself to self-citation:

> Outreplus, comme l'experience fait mieux entendre un faict, ce n'est point sans cause que Dieu en sa Loy menaçant son peuple s'il ne luy obeit de luy envoyer la famine, dit expressement qu'il fera que l'homme tendre et delicat, c'est à dire d'un naturel autrement doux et bening, et qui auparavant avoit choses cruelles en horreur, en l'extremité de la famine deviendra neantmoins si desnaturé qu'en regardant son prochain, voire sa femme et ses enfans d'un mauvais oeil, il appetera d'en manger. Car outre les exemples que j'ay narrez en l'histoire de Sancerre, tant du pere et de la mere qui mangerent de leur propre enfant, que de quelques soldats, lesquels ayans essayé de la chair des corps humains qui avoyent esté tuez en guerre, ont confessé depuis que si l'affliction eust encores continué, ils estoyent en deliberation de se ruer sur les vivans. (*Histoire d'un voyage,* 535–36/212–13)

> Furthermore, as experience makes a fact better understood, one comprehends why it is that God, in the Book of Deuteronomy [28.53–54], threatening to send his people to famine if they do not obey him, says expressly that the man who is tender and delicate, that is, of a gentle and benign nature, and who formerly had a horror of cruel things, in the

extremity of famine will nevertheless become so denatured that he will look with an evil eye upon his neighbor, even his wife and his children, and desire to eat them. In the history of Sancerre I have recounted the examples of father and mother who ate their own child, and of some soldiers who tasted the flesh of human bodies that had been killed in war, and who have confessed since that if the affliction had continued, they would have hurled themselves upon the living.

As Frank Lestringant mentions, Léry returns to the same passage in his emotional opening, of the depiction of cannibalism committed by the Potard family, but it is less of a psychological explanation of the cruel and desperate transformation in human beings than an exclamatory preparation for the events to follow.[17] The immediacy of the horror—that human beings brought up to hold such cruel acts in abhorrence should disobey God's Law—does not allow the narrator in this earlier work to engage in an expanded exploration of the moral effect of hunger.

On board ship on the return voyage from Brazil, Léry makes it very clear, as he had in referencing the majority of the Huguenots in Sancerre, that he and his men restrained from desperate actions in the face of extreme hunger because of their fear of God: "Je puis asseurer veritablement, que durant nostre famine sur mer, nous estions si chagrins qu'encores que nous fussions retenus par la crainte de Dieu, à peine pouvions nous parler l'un à l'autre sans nous fascher" (*Histoire d'un voyage faict en la terre du Brésil*, 536/213) [I can testify that during our famine on the sea we were so despondent and irritable that although we were restrained by the fear of God, so we could scarcely speak to each other without getting angry]. They were not exempt from "barbarous thoughts regarding barbarous acts" ("mauvaises volontez touchant cest acte barbare"). For these Christians—"ceux de la religion," as Léry would often call the Huguenots—it is a question of will ("volonté") in resisting hunger and basing action on the fear of God. Yet temptation is a part of the human experience and has been since the fall of humankind. Such is the lesson of these two *Histoires*. It is not human strength but the spirit of God flowing through individuals, and through the narrator of these two accounts, that allows the Huguenots to persist in spite of persecution and lies.

As I conclude this analysis of cannibalism within the context of Léry's *Histoire mémorable du siège de Sancerre* and *Histoire d'un voyage faict en la terre du Brésil*, let me look to the final passages of both works in order to show that the former work is one in which, for the most part, Léry's key role is that of witness to the harshness of the siege, the bravery of the besieged, and the inspiration and strength that flowed through them from God. In the second work, he is more aware of his role as chronicler, more conscious of rhetorical conventions, such as the modesty topos, and equally engaged yet more persistent in his condemnation of his Catholic rivals Thevet and Villegagnon—figures that are not central to the history of the siege of Sancerre. The story of the siege of Sancerre was written quickly, while the Brazilian chronicle benefitted from the time Léry spent reflecting upon the events and from the time taken in the composition of the work.

The cruel death of three figures hangs over the final chapter of the *Histoire mémorable du siège de Sancerre*. First, there is the massacre of the bailiff Johanneau, the elected leader of Sancerre, who was tricked by the besiegers into thinking that La Châtre wanted to see him. En route, they tell him he is going to die. He begs for time to ask the Lord to forgive his sins, and before he has finished, the soldiers massacre him with dagger thrusts ("à coups de dagues"). Léry leaves us the portrait of the martyrdom—Johanneau praying with such zeal that the murderers confessed subsequently that they had never heard anyone speak better nor pray to God in such a way ("Pria d'un tel zele et d'une telle affection, que les meurtriers qui le tenoyent e entendoyent, ont confessé depuis, qu il s n'avoyent jamais oüy mieux parler, ny prier Dieu de telle sorte"; 339).

Two other figures, Pierre de la Bourgade, Minister of God's Word, and his wife, are shot by a soldier. Yet the most pitiful figure is the widow of Johanneau—throwing herself on her knees before La Châtre, who lies to her about the fate of her husband. The final portrait of the widow Johanneau is of an impoverished woman who has lost her belongings, her husband, and her money through the cruelty of the besiegers. She is a symbol of the habitants of Sancerre, "demeurez appovris" (342). The besiegers' reduction of Sancerre to nothing—by removing town clocks, church bells, and other distinguishing town markers—is summed up in Léry's phrase, written in all capital letters: "ICY FUT SANCERRE." The finality of the historic past tense noted in the use of the *passé simple* ("fut") highlights the brutality of temporal actions taken against the besieged. These are material things, but the deprivation extends to the spiritual domain, when their church is taken from the inhabitants of Sancerre ("par la ruine et dissipation de leur Eglise") to be replaced by idolatry and papal superstitions ("l'idolatrie, et les supersitions Papales"; 342). To convey the enormity of this final act, in addition to all the other cruelties, Léry returns to the image of cannibalism and gives the practice a figurative twist as he describes the ferocity with which the Catholic forces dealt with the

Huguenots at the end of the siege: "on achevera de succer le sang et la moëlle" (342) [they finished off by sucking the blood and the marrow].[18]

Léry concludes his account of the siege not just by blaming the cruelty of the Catholic soldiers and leaders but also by condemning the scorn of God's grace ("mespris des graces de Dieu") along with that cursed greed ("ceste maudite avarice"; 343). Without returning to his own role in recounting the suffering caused by the siege, Léry ends with an appeal for human charity and a critique of those who have refused to help their "povres freres" by giving "un sol à Dieu" and thus inciting God's wrath. But he recognizes that it is up to God, so accustomed to ruining his enemies by causing his children to suffer, to take pity on "son povre peuple, et de son Eglise Françoise," in name of Jesus Christ (*Histoire mémorable du siège de Sancerre*, 343). The invocation to the Lord on behalf of the sins of all those in Sancerre and throughout France reflects his role as witness, effaced before the Lord. He exhibits the humility mentioned in the previous chapter of this book in relation to Saint Augustine's concept of the Christus medicus. The willingness to humble oneself before Christ, a trait cited by the Catholic poet Ronsard in his rebuke of Huguenot Brother Zamariel, is a critical element of faith.

The self-effacement noted above is not present in the concluding remarks of the *Histoire d'un voyage faict en la terre du Brésil*. After strongly condemning Villegagnon for chastising "de bouche et par escrit Ceux de la religion" and for being the first to shed the blood of the children of God in this newly discovered land ("le premier qui a respandu le sand des enfans de Dieu en ce pays nouvellement cogneu"; 549/218), Léry goes on to speak of Villegagnon's resumption of his Catholic ways— in the order of Malta and his death. He showed the same disregard for his relatives as he had for the Huguenot ministers who came to help him in Brazil.

Léry devotes the remaining paragraphs not to witnessing the travails of those of his religion, but to describing his own experience. He explains how he faced death many times and so had come to know firsthand "that it is the Eternal who causes us to live and to die, to descend into the grave and to arise from it" (I Samuel 2:6). While he is still invoking the scripture and the infinite goodness of God for coming to his rescue many times, he is the recipient of God's mercy. The focus is on Léry and on his observations: "C'est finalement, ce que j'ay observé, tant sur mer en allant et retournant en la terre du Brésil dite Amerique, que parmi les sauvages habitans audit pays" (*Histoire d'un voyage*, 551/219) [That, finally, is what I have observed, both on the sea, during the voyage to and from the land of Brazil, called America, and among the savages who live in that country].

There follows an apology for his style—as if he has suddenly become aware of narrative conventions of the modesty topos: "Je sçay bien toutesfois qu'ayant si beau sujet je n'ay pas traité les diverses matieres que j'ay touchées, d'un tel style ni d'une façon si grave qu'il falloit" (551/219) [I know, however, that having such a fine subject, I have not treated the various matters that I have mentioned in a style or a manner as grave as was required]. He apologizes for either overemphasizing something that could have been treated more briefly or not spending enough time on other topics. Both Lestringant's edition and Janet Whatley's translation use the second edition as a base for their work, with ample notes to other editions. Léry in this 1580 edition notes that it is a second edition, and tips his hat to his readers and hopes that they will pardon his "defauts du langage" (551/219).

Of his concluding remarks, only the last sentence recalls the concluding paragraphs of his previous work, the *Histoire mémorable du siège de Sancerre.* He gives a sort of benediction: "Or au Roy des siecles immortel et invisible, à Dieu seul sage soit honneur et gloire eternellement, Amen" (552/219) [Now to the King of the Ages, immortal and invisible, to God who alone is wise, be all honor and glory, world without end. Amen]. Praising not the mortal, temporal kings of Europe, but the immortal King, he brings his work back into the atemporal world that one remembers from his account of the siege of Sancerre—where the suffering and punishment recall the times of persecution from the Old Testament as well as other sieges in human experience across time. The painful imagery and emptiness evoked in the conclusion to his account of the siege and the effaced presence of the narrator/witness have given way to the author/narrator being eager to connect with his readers as they make their way through this and subsequent editions of his work. Yet, the image of cannibalism, the abundant cross-references to each of the two *Histoires,* and the self-citation will forever lead readers to remember both works and to link them together in the struggle for "ceux de la religion" to find a space to practice their religion and to experience freedom of conscience.

The Old World Meets the New in Montaigne's *Essais*

Syphilis, Cannibalism, and Empirical Medicine

THE LAST DECADE of the fifteenth century brought an unusual conjunction of discovery, warfare, and medical science to spotlight the arrival of what since the eighteenth century has been called syphilis. The disease was known by the Italians as the *mal francese* or by physicians as the *morbus gallicus* for the connection made between the invasion of Naples in 1494 and the eventual conquest by the French under Charles VIII.[1] The French attributed the disease's origins to an epidemic emanating from Naples: poisoned water, "vengeful Spaniards mixing leper's blood with wine" (Eamon, 5). Each nation preferred to blame the other for introducing a new infection.

The chronicles coming back from the New World soon placed the blame outside Europe and tied the new pandemic to inhabitants of the New World: Gonzalo Fernández de Oviedo y Valdes, Bartolomé de las Casas, and Ruy Diaz de Isla.[2] Eamon points out that "blaming the other is one possible response to new diseases. Another is to blame oneself" (Eamon, 2). The focus of this chapter is Michel de Montaigne's interest in the chronicles of the explorers of the New World to shed light on conflict and bloodshed in Europe. Montaigne will use the vocabulary of sickness and disease to reflect upon contrasts between the Old and the New World. To do so, he appropriates some of the rhetoric of one of

Italy's most controversial medical spokespersons—Leonardo Fioravanti (1517–1588)—and yet sets himself in sharp opposition to the charlatan's practices. That Montaigne was aware of Fioravanti's medical pronouncements and practices is known from "De la ressemblance des enfans aux peres" [Of the Resemblance of Children to Fathers].³ Here, Montaigne mentions the innovations introduced—often at the peril of the patient—by "Paraclese, Fioravanti et Argenterius" (II: 37, 772A/586).

Montaigne and Fioravanti were both proponents of the empiricists when it came to medicine. The experience gained by the patient in suffering the disease outstrips scientific knowledge. For Montaigne, "L'experience est proprement sur son fumier au subject de la medecine, où la raison luy quite toute la place" (III: 13, 1079B/826) [Experience is really on its own dunghill in the subject of medicine, where reason yields it the whole field]. He agrees with Plato that to be a true physician and accurate diagnostician, one needs to have experienced all the sicknesses that one seeks to remedy, and he adds syphilis to the list: "C'est raison qu'ils prennent la verole s'ils la veulent sçavoir penser" (III: 13, 1079B/827) [It is reasonable that he should catch the pox if he wants to know how to treat it]. In the sixteenth century, syphilis was never far from any discussion of disease (*lues*) or epidemic, just as in the late twentieth century, AIDS dominated both lay and scientific medical discussions. Accurate diagnosis and treatment demands risk taking, and the physician willing to experience illness in order to treat it more effectively is the only doctor Montaigne would trust: "Vrayment je m'en fierois à celuy là." The others are like artists, safely inside illustrating the treacherous seas and shoals outside or building a model ship without encountering any risk: "Car les autres nous guident comme celuy qui peint les mers, les escueils et les ports, estant assis sur sa table et y faict promener le modèle d'un navire en toute seureté" (III: 13, 1079/827). In another essay, while not claiming profound medical knowledge beyond his observation of his own bouts of illness, he acknowledges that his youthful amorous inclinations, which he calls "erreurs de sa jeunesse," led him to ignore the dangers he might encounter and to experience the first symptoms of venereal disease without lasting effect: "deux atteintes legeres toutesfois et preambulaires" ("De trois commerces," III: 3, 826C/627). It is indeed noteworthy that the discussion of his sexually contracted disease was added in the Bordeaux copy, as the essayist expands the detailed medical descriptions of the final essays, to be discussed further on in the present chapter. Antonia Szabari notes that Montaigne proposes, in "De l'art de conferer," to present his "erreurs" to his readers as cautionary tales, just as the wheels of justice condemn transgressors as a way to warn others: "Publiant et accusant mes imperfections, quelqu'un apprendra à les craindre" (III: 8, 822B/703) [By my publishing and accusing my imperfections, someone will learn to fear them].[4] Ronsard had made a similar "public confession" ("Or je veux que ma vie en escrit apparoisse"; *Oeuvres complètes,* II: 606, v. 22) in his "Response aux injures et calomnies" when he spoke about his pleasure in the company of women, amid other tasks such as study, writing, prayer, and walks in nature (*Oeuvres complètes,* II: 607, n. 18). As they offer up their lives and their daily routine for scrutiny, two self-avowed Catholic authors give a nod toward the public admission of their deeds. Montaigne, like Ronsard before him, knows the value of observing a person's habits in taking the measure of an individual.

Montaigne makes it clear that three generations of his family—all suffering from kidney stones—shared a scorn for medical practices. "Que les medecins excusent un peu ma liberté, car, par cette mesme infusion et insinuation fatale, j'ay receu la haine et le mespris de leur doctrine" (II: 37, 764A/579) [Let the doctors excuse my liberty a bit, for by this same fatal infusion and insinuation I have received my hatred and contempt for their teaching]. He reinforces the superiority of experience to science: "La medecine se forme par exemples et experience; aussi faict mon opinion" (764A/579) [Medicine is based on examples and experience; so is my opinion]. The movement and undulation that typify medical practice in the specific context of the individual echo the fluctuation and change that characterize Montaigne's own writing. Medicine and writing share the characteristic that they are both a snapshot in time—framed by the circumstances surrounding the moment of application. It is here that Montaigne and Fioravanti diverge, but also here that they converge on a topic that will intrigue both of them: cannibalism.

Eamon notes that Fioravanti's "work also carried a theoretical and ideological message: it was about the failure of 'scientific' medicine and the value of experience over theory, the veracity of people's wisdom, the worth of 'natural' ways of healing, and above all the importance to physicians of sagacity and good judgment which can be gained only by long experience in the ways of nature" (Eamon, 10). For Fioravanti, disease is the result of a "corruption of the body caused by unnatural conduct" (Eamon, 10). The cure for the disease is a remedy that ultimately causes the expulsion of the "bodily corruption" (Eamon, 10). Montaigne abhorred such violent therapies applied by physicians to the patient—

remedies that "rendent la santé malade" (II: 37, 766A/581) [make health sick]. Without the help of doctors, he found his illnesses "douces à supporter" (766A/581) [easy to endure].

Fioravanti made a name for himself in the treatment of syphilis based on a series of "drugs that purged the body of 'pollutions'" (Eamon, 16). He prescribed "sarsaparilla to induce vomiting" and had "an armory of emetics and purgatives" (Eamon, 16). These were precisely the type of violent cures decried by Montaigne: remedies that broke the daily diet and habits of the patient. Calling upon his own experience and that of his father and grandfather, he states that "ma forme de vie est pareille en maladie comme en santé: mesme lict, mesmes heures, mesmes viandes me servent, et mesme breuvage" (III: 13, 1080B/827) [My way of life is the same in sickness as in health; the same bed, the same hours, the same food serve me, and the same drink].

Given their different approaches to treating disease, why would Montaigne have noticed Fioravanti's medical writings? Taking his notion that disease is the result of bodily corruption, Fioravanti links syphilis to cannibalism, but his theory runs counter to the views of Oviedo and Las Casas, who saw syphilis as a new disease originating in the New World. For Fioravanti it is an old disease and results—as do all diseases, in his view—from bodily corruption.[5] In this instance, syphilis resulted from the cooking practices of the camp cooks of the soldiers in Naples during the French invasion. Short of food, cooks of both armies "secretly took the flesh of the dead" for use in a variety of dishes served to the soldiers (Eamon, 10). This led Fioravanti to experiment in feeding animals chopped-up parts of their own species to see whether the symptoms of syphilis would appear. He claimed that the pustules and fever characteristic of the disease showed up on those animals who had eaten pieces of their own kind. For the surgeon, this was proof that syphilis was the result of corrupt practice—the unnatural act of eating one's own species (Eamon, 17).

The chronicles of Oviedo, Las Casas, André Thevet (*Les Singularités de la France Antarctique*), and Jean de Léry (*Histoires d'un voyage faict en la terre du Brésil*) had captured the imagination of the Europeans. The proponents of the Counter-Reformation used the reports of cannibalism among the indigenous peoples of the New World as evidence that they were less than human and so could be enslaved and maltreated. Eamon cites Anthony Pagdon's view that consuming human flesh was considered a violation of natural law prohibiting the eating of one's own kind.[6] Montaigne follows most closely the account of cannibalistic practice reported by the Protestant chronicler Jean de Léry, and as I have pointed out elsewhere, Léry's power of observation was much like that of the modern anthropologist.[7] He wanted to detail and comprehend the customs within the cultural context. Montaigne understood that cannibalism in the context of Tupinamba society was a cultural practice, not a flesh-eating orgy or something done to appease hunger. Dudley D. Marchi comments, "The practice of Tupinamba anthropophagy . . . interpreted by Montaigne, following Léry, is a sign which unifies their community: a practice of collective ritual, an economy of tribal presence, preservation, and self-identification."[8] As noted in the previous chapter, Montaigne observes: "Ce n'est pas, comme on pense, pour s'en nourrir, ainsi que faisoient anciennement les Scythes: c'est pour representer une extreme vengeance" (I: 31, 209A/155) [This is not, as people think, for nourishment, as of old the Scythians used to do; it is to betoken an extreme revenge]. He sets the courage and valor of the Tupinamba in sharp moral contrast to the pusillanimity of the Portuguese in the New World, who buried the Indians waist-deep and then pulled on their appendages before hanging them. The essayist is troubled by the Europeans' failure to see value in the customs of the Indians: "Je ne suis pas marry que nous remerquons l'horreur barbaresque qu'il y a en une telle action, mais ouy bien dequoy, jugeans bien de leurs fautes, nous soyons si aveuglez aux nostres" (209A/155) [I am not sorry that we notice the barbarous horror of such acts, but I am heartily sorry that, judging their faults rightly, we should be so blind to our own]. Here Montaigne gets to the heart of why he has seized on cannibalism to make a moral point:

> Je pense qu'il y a plus de barbarie à manger un homme vivant qu'à le manger mort, à deschirer, par tourmens et par geénes, un corps encore plein de sentiment, le faire rostir par le menu, le faire mordre et meurtrir aux chiens et aux pourceaux (comme nous l'avons, non seulement leu mais veu de fresche memoire, non entre des ennemis anciens, mais entre des voisins et concitoyens, et, qui pis est, sous pretexte de piété et de religion), que de le rostir et manger apres qu'il est trespassé. (209A/155).
>
> I think there is more barbarity in eating a man alive than in eating him dead; and in tearing by tortures and the rack a body still full of feeling, in roasting a man bit by bit, in having him bitten and mangled by dogs and swine (as we have not only read but seen within fresh memory, not

among ancient enemies, but among neighbors and fellow citizens, and what is worse, on the pretext of piety and religion), than in roasting and eating him after he is dead.

Cannibalism became a way to focus on religion and cultural practice—but in diverting attention away from Europe to the New World, the subject was less controversial. Description of the ritualistic practice, consuming a piece of the flesh not for sustenance but to punish the enemy, combined with the details on housing, drink, marriage, warfare, and prophets, distracted the reader from the political and religious controversies in the Old World. But soon the mirror reflected back on the Old World and its savage treatment of neighbors and countrymen persecuted for their religious views. Cannibalism became a signifier for things gone awry in the Old World. In fact, Frank Lestringant shows how the valiant death song of the prisoner of the indigenous Brazilians parallels the controversy over transubstantiation in the Europe, a major dispute in the violent wars of religion.

> Ces muscles, dit-il, cette cher et ces veines, ce sont les vostres, pauvres fols que vous estes; vous ne recognoissez pas la substance des membres de vos ancestres. (*Les Essais*, I: 31, 212A/158)

> "These muscles," he says, "this flesh and these veins are your own, poor fools that you are. You do not recognize that the substance of your ancestors' limbs is still contained in them."

Lestringant mentions Montaigne's audacity in creating a parallel between the Tupi prisoner and Christ. Their bodies, consumed in ritual celebration, will be a reminder of the valiance and sacrifice with which they lived (Lestringant, *Une Sainte horreur*, 296–98). It is as if in constructing such a daring parallel, the essayist laments the absence of valor of the populace at home and the reliance on "soldats empruntez," or mercenary soldiers (III: 12, 1042B/796).

Montaigne, taking a cue from Léry, looks to the New World—the Tupinamba—for a remedy for what has failed in Europe: "Les loix naturelles leur commandent encores, fort peu abastardies par les nostres" (I: 31, 206A/153) [The laws of nature still rule them, very little corrupted by ours]. Europe has not yet spread its contagion—its unnatural laws—to the New World. In fact, the Tupinamba live in a temperate climate that preserves their health: there is no talk of syphilis, no mention of doctors, no need for physicians since they are rarely sick. Montaigne points out that the discovery of the New World has introduced new remedies—these very natural remedies known to the indigenous people. Europeans went all the way across the ocean—pulled by the appeal of what is exotic and rare—in pursuit of these remedies: "le gayac, la salseperille et le bois desquine" (II: 37, 772A/585) [guaiacum, sarsaparilla, and chinaroot].

The mention of natural remedies and sarsaparilla brings me back to Fioravanti—a man who blurred the distinction between surgeon (limited to external treatments) and physician (credentialed to treat patients internally). Fioravanti rose to medical visibility by using a natural remedy, sarsaparilla—a remedy known by the indigenous people of the New World—to treat syphilis. His treatment of syphilis relied on drugs that purged the body of "pollutions." He prescribed sarsaparilla to induce vomiting and followed up with "a decoction of *legno santo*" (Eamon, 16). Eamon speaks of a kind of "physiological exorcism": "His treatments, acts of purification, mimicked the exorcist's rite of chasing away the demons from tormented bodies" (Eamon, 20).

In performing experiments to show that syphilis could indeed have spread from cutting up human bodies to feed to invading and resident armies in Naples, Fioravanti attributed the outbreak of a pandemic to a moral lapse in the body politic. "Fioravanti believed that the cause of Italy's moral and political decline was an internal pollution that began with the courts and spread outward to contaminate the entire commonwealth" (Eamon, 20). His *Capricci medicinali* indicates that he urged princes to ignore flatterers: "just as the 'bad quality of the stomach' spreads its contagion to all the body's organs, so corrupt rulers and their fawning courtiers ruined the whole body politic."[9]

Fioravanti adhered to the perspective of the Catholics, who decried the rise of evangelical Christianity and the rise of Protestantism. Yet what is striking here is that he found positive things to say about the medical practices of the indigenous peoples of the New World: "He credited the Indian shamans with numerous discoveries, including not only a host of medicaments unknown to the Europeans but also a certain herb that enabled them to see into the future" (Eamon, 22). Like Montaigne, he challenged the established view that the cannibals were without science. "Moreover, he turned the conventional blame system inside-out, attributing the onset of syphilis in Europe not to the Indians, but to the barbarous behavior of the Europeans themselves."[10]

Both empiricists, Montaigne and Fioravanti blamed current conventional medical practices, advanced by scientific experimentation rather than by sound consultation with the patient. Spurred on by a more "natural" approach, they commented on the herbal remedies that even academic physicians were acquiring at great expense and danger: "au hasard d'une si longue peregrination et si perilleuse" (*Les Essais,* II: 37, 772A/586).

It is important to note that their approaches were drastically different. Fioravanti favored violent natural remedies that purged the body of impurities, while Montaigne resisted medical treatment that might interrupt the "douce" unfolding of daily habit. Yet, they both saw virtue in the established practices of the inhabitants of the New World and attributed barbarous actions to the corrupt leaders of Europe. The common signifier is cannibalism at home. The common link is syphilis, or at least the common remedy, sarsaparilla—seen as one remedy in the toolbox of "natural" medicines used by the indigenous shamans in the New World with greater efficacy than was shown by the learned physicians of the Old World. The coincidence of the outbreak of syphilis, the French invasion of Naples, and the return of Columbus's crew from the New World led the Europeans to pin the blame for the pandemic on a remote source: the native peoples of the New World. "Placing blame for such catastrophic occurrences defines the normal, establishes the boundaries of appropriate behavior, and isolates the cause of fear" (Eamon, 21).

As I have noted earlier, Fioravanti and Montaigne both looked to experience in seeking knowledge about sickness. Three generations of the essayist's family spurned medical care: "Mes ancestres avoient la medecine à contrecoeur par quelque inclination occulte et naturelle: car la veuë mesme des drogues faisoit horreur à mon pere" (II: 37, 764A/579) [My ancestors had an aversion to medicine by some occult natural inclination: for the very sight of drugs filled my father with horror]. Fioravanti's antipathy for scientific medicine as opposed to empirical medicine came from practical experience in seeing the "physicians" scorn observation and remedies handed down through the "non-scientific" or folk practitioners. "Rejecting the abstruseness of modern medicine, Fioravanti urged a return to the pristine and simple methods of the 'first physicians,' who had no medical system or scientific method, but just used good judgment" (Eamon, 15). As Eamon points out, the "first cause" of all ailment originates in the stomach—hence the need to purge the stomach violently and frequently from whatever was causing impurities (Eamon, 15). One of the drawbacks of the empiricists is that they look for symptoms instead of for the overall picture of the disease. The empiricist doctor studies symptoms of individual patients (Eamon, 17). While Montaigne would decry the violent purges promoted by such drastic medical practitioners as Fioravanti, the attention Fioravanti paid to an individual's response to the disease and to medication would resonate with the essayist. His observation in later life of his own youthful experience with venereal disease—"deux atteintes, legeres, toutesfois et preambulaires"—is a case in point (III: 3, 826C/627).

One of the virtues of Eamon's work on Fioravanti is that he makes the link between Fioravanti's medical views of the individual body, or microcosm, and extends them to his view of the body politic. To do so, he cites the anthropologist Mary Douglas: "There is a continual exchange of meanings between the two kinds of bodily experience so that each reinforces the categories of the other."[11] Eamon goes on to state that "Fioravanti's conception of the body as a physiological system that was vulnerable to various contaminations mirrored his conception of society as a moral order narrowly teetering on the balance between purity and corruption" (Eamon, 21).

Two historic events coincided: the exploration of the New World, with the subsequent awareness of cannibalism and syphilis, and the outbreak of the Wars of Religion, followed by acts of extreme violence and extreme vengeance. Douglas shows how the language of pandemic was applied to the body politic, as the physical body and the body politic became conflated (discussed by Eamon, 21). With increasing fervor as the three books unfold and as his additions to the *Essais* lead the readers to focus on the impact of intolerance, corruption, and violence on the society, Montaigne transfers the metaphor of illness to the body politic. Contemporary to the growing violence of the Wars of Religion is his individual struggle with kidney stones. The language of his individual physical struggle spills over to describe the ills of France. One might ask if Montaigne latched on to the medical language and the image of cannibalism in order to tone down a more incendiary political language or whether he drew a parallel between his own declining health and the health of the state. By the final chapters of Book III of the *Essais,* he has made the commitment to address the political corruption openly, and yet the medical metaphors, used to address his own observation of his medical condition as well as the state of the body politic, have become part of the fiber of his discourse. Ronsard had already depicted France as a deathly ill woman with frightful hair and deep, recessed eyes: "une pauvre femme attainte de la mort"; "son poil estoit hideux, son oeil have et profond" ("Continuation du discours des miseres de ce temps"; *Oeuvres complètes,* II: 557, vv. 15, 18). So Montaigne is not alone in expanding the medical metaphor to include the body politic. A comparison of "Des cannibales" (Book I) with "Des coches," "De la phisionomie," and "De l'experience" (Book III) demonstrates the increasing intensity of the application of the medical metaphor to the body politic.

Mention of medicine is rare in "Des cannibales." It begins with an analogy between the feverish movements of the sick body and those of the geographical landscape that changed the shape of Montaigne's Dordogne River: "Il semble qu'il y aye des mouvemens, naturels les uns, les autres fievreux, en ces grands corps comme aux nostres" (I: 31, 204B and C/151) [It seems that there are movements, some natural, other feverish, in these great bodies, just as in our own]. The next allusion to sickness is to the fact that the Tupinamba are rarely ill: "Il est rare d'y voir un homme malade; et m'ont asseuré n'en y avoir veu aucun tremblant, chassieux, edenté, ou cour bé de vieillesse" (207A/153) [It is rare to see a sick man there; and they have assured me that they never saw one palsied, bleary-eyed, toothless, or bent with age]. Montaigne here subscribes to the idea that the natural remedies and the healthy lifestyle contribute to keeping the inhabitants of the New World healthier than their European counterparts. The final reference to medicine in this essay is to the audacity of physicians to try all sorts of remedies on their patients—remedies as extreme as the efforts of Montaigne's ancestors to survive Caesar's siege of the town of Alésia by feeding the more resilient townspeople the remains of the feeble: "Et les medecins ne craignent pas de s'en servir à toute sorte d'usage pour nostre santé, soit pour l'appliquer au dedans ou au dehors; mais il ne se trouva jamais aucune opinion si desreglée qui excusat la trahison, la desloyauté, la tyrannie, la cruauté, qui sont nos fautes ordinaires" (210A/156) [And physicians do not fear to use human flesh in all sorts of ways for our health, applying it either inwardly or outwardly. But there never was any opinion so disordered as to excuse treachery, disloyalty, tyranny, and cruelty, which are our ordinary vices]. Cannibalism is not unknown in Europe; it is not confined to the "other," the "barbaric" inhabitants of the New World.

The final chapter in Book II of the *Essais*, "De la ressemblance des enfans aux peres," is devoted to medicine. As I have stated above, Montaigne evokes the antipathy in which his father, grandfather, and other members of his family have held the medical arts. He also notes that while he is not subject to the suffering that touches our soul, he is vulnerable to physical pain: "Mais les souffrances vrayment essentielles et corporelles, je les gouste bien vifvement" (II: 37, 760A/575) [But the really essential and bodily sufferings I feel very keenly]. This chapter takes medical science to task: "En premier lieu, l'experience me le fait craindre: car, de ce que j'ay de connoissance, je ny voy nulle race de gens si tost malade et si tard guerie que celle qui est sous la jurisidiction de la medicine" (766A/581) [In the first place, experience makes me fear it; for as far as my knowledge goes, I see no group of people so soon sick and so late cured as those who are under the jurisdiction of medicine]. He speaks of gentle experience when he does not have to suffer the bitter remedies of the medical establishment, "l'amertume de leurs ordonnances" (766/581). Intrusive medical practice disrupts the normal flow of life.

The only remedy that he continues to experience is the beneficial effects of the natural mineral baths: "Voilà comment cette partie de medecine à laquelle seule je me suis laissé aller, quoy qu'elle soit la moins artificielle, si a elle sa bonne part de la confusion et incertitude qui se voit par tout ailleurs en cet art" (777A/590–91) [Thus you see how this part of medicine, to which alone I have abandoned myself, although it is the least artificial, still has its good share of the confusion and uncertainty that is seen everywhere else in this art]. Montaigne makes it clear that he has known some worthy doctors and that his antipathy is for the medical arts: "Ce n'est pas à eux que j'en veux, c'est à leur art" (780A/593) [My quarrel is not with them but with their art]. Along with the hot baths, Montaigne gives some credence to folk remedies: "Il n'est pas une simple femmelette de qui n'employons les barbotages et les brevets; et, selon mon humeur, si j'avoy à en accepter quelqu'une, j'accepterois plus volontiers cette medecine qu'aucune autre, d'autant qu'aumoins il n'y a nul dommage à craindre" (781A/593) [There is not the simplest little woman whose mumblings and magic formulas we do not employ; and for my taste, if I had to take any, I would accept this medicine more willingly than any other, inasmuch as at least there is no harm to be feared from it]. Montaigne is not far from the teachings of Paracelsus, who "exempted from his blanket condemnation [of physicians and apothecaries] . . . those who relied on 'experience and personal practice.'"[12]

Jean Starobinski has brilliantly demonstrated that in criticizing the medical profession, Montaigne frequently echoes the form and content of medical discourse.[13] In following the manner in which Montaigne describes his body and his illness in the essay "De l'experience," Starobinski remarks: "The reader will notice (were he only to glance at the medical books of the time) that Montaigne cannot narrate his own being (*se raconter*) except by appropriating the language of the doctors, by *making use* of their categories, by diverting them, according to the rule he applies to all of his borrowings, for his own benefit" (Starobinski, 279–80).

Abrupt change in habit that is a part of the scientific medical art is the target of Montaigne's critique. Effective remedies were best harvested in the climates in which the patients lived in order to avoid disrupting the natural routine. In 1533, Symphorien Champier urged "the French to find remedies for all their illnesses in France, not to bring over medicines from foreign sources."[14] In his essay "De la ressemblance des enfans aux peres" (II: 37), Montaigne interweaves the medical history of his family—his grandfather, his father, and himself—with the history of medicine. Here again, his discourse reflects the discourse of medical humanists of his time. One particular reference, to guaiac wood, links the topic of cannibalism, the story of the indigenous populations of the New World, to syphilis and medicine. Montaigne echoes the views of his contemporary medical writers, such as Paracelsus and Champier, in railing against the importation of exotic remedies from the New World: "Si les nations desquelles nous retirons le gayac, la salseperille et le bois desquine, ont des medecins, combien pensons nous, par cette mesme recommandation de l'estrangeté, la rareté et la cherté, qu'ils facent feste de nos choux et de nostre persil: car qui oseroit mespriser les choses recherchées de si loing . . . ?" (II: 37, 772A/585–86) [If the countries from which we get guaiacum, sarsaparilla, and chinaroot have doctors, how much, we may imagine, through this same recommendation of strangeness, rarity, and costliness, must they prize our cabbages and our parsley! For who would dare despise things sought out at such a distance, at the risk of such a long and perilous voyage?]. The explorers had brought back these much-touted remedies. "One of the earliest of these, guaiac wood from the Andes, was reputed to cure the new 'French pox' and thus easily attracted swarms of buyers and sellers, wheelers and dealers" (Cooper, 34). In the very same instance that he is echoing a view of Paracelsus in preferring homegrown remedies to those sought from afar, Montaigne attacks the medical practice of the likes of "Paracelse, Fioravanti and Argenterius" for changing established practice too often without providing time for the patient to adapt to new prescriptions: "car ils ne changent pas seulement une recepte, mais, à ce qu'on me dict, toute la contexture et police du corps de la medecine, accusant d'ignorance et de piperie ceux qui n ont faict profesion jusques à eux" (II: 37, 772A/586) [for they change not merely one prescription, but, so they tell me, the whole contexture and order of the body of medicine, accusing of ignorance or deception all who have professed it before them]. The patient is left to adapt and suffer. Better to try out the more inexact science of folk remedies or thermal cures that do no harm than to submit to the perilous innovations of medical science.[15]

Montaigne's family rejected the notion that they should yield their experience with their illness, their familiarity with their individual situation, to the "savoir" of the university-trained physicians. It was a case of "connoissance" over "savoir," familiarity over innovation (Starobinski, 278). In preferring long-established home remedies and therapeutic baths found in proximity over drugs that hailed from exotic places, Montaigne, and some of his contemporary physicians and medical writers, was conflating the body with the body politic. National provenance mattered, if only because the body was better served from remedies that were found close at hand. Borrowing from Brunfels, who called for seeking German herbs and remedies, Champier "enjoined his readers to recognize their true identity—'We're in Celtic France, amidst Christians'—and advised his readers that since they were 'Christians, not Muslims' 'French, not Arabs, or Egyptians, or those born in India or Palestine,' what they really needed to preserve their health were locally-grown medicinals."[16] Emerging national identity took the form of religion, crops, cooking, and climate.

With the third book of essays, Montaigne's bitterness against the violence to humankind grows as the French Wars of Religion come even closer to home and set neighbor against neighbor, brother against brother. While medicine plays only a minor role in "Des coches," the vehemence of Montaigne's attack on European inhumanity shown to the indigenous people of Mexico and Peru escalates. The title of the essay, "Des coches," reveals Montaigne's physical weakness in getting sick while traveling in coaches, litters, or boats, and serves to conceal the true topic of the essay, the inhumane treatment of the indigenous people of Mexico and Peru as well as the intellectual, moral, and physical superiority of these people. Medical doctors have counseled the essayist to wrap a towel around his stomach to ward off seasickness or the upset stomach that comes with riding in a carriage or litter. He would rather overcome such physical weakness through his own moral courage—a sort of natural response to personal defect: "Les medecins m'ont ordonné de me presser et sangler d'une serviette le bas du ventre pour remedier à cet accident; ce que je n'ay point essayé, ayant accoutumé de luicter les deffauts qui sont en moy et les dompter par moy-mesme" (III: 6, 901B/687) [The doctors have ordered me to bind and swathe my abdomen with a towel to remedy this trouble; which I have not tried, being accustomed to wrestle with the weaknesses that are in me and overcome them by myself].

He proceeds to illustrate the cowardly, dishonest treatment of the indigenous people by the Spanish and Portuguese in the name of the king and in the name of religion. The presumption of the Europeans has already proven deceptive in that while they claimed to have invented gunpowder and moveable type, it was a false claim because the Chinese had discovered both innovations a thousand years before, in "un autre bout du monde" (III: 6, 908B/693) [in another corner of the world]. Europe refuses to acknowledge that the inhabitants of either "bout du monde"—the representative "other"—could have acquired scientific knowledge. It was by ruse and deception that the Europeans managed to overcome the people of Mexico and Peru. Absent the surprise effect of the arrival of horses and gunpowder used to overwhelm the Mexicans and Tupinamba, "vous leur ostez toute l'occasion de tant de victoires" (910B/694) [eliminate this disparity . . . and you take from the conquerors the whole basis of so many victories]. What is quite remarkable, if one removes the context in which Montaigne sets his description of the courage and valor of the native peoples of the New World, is that the essayist could be referring to Jews and Protestants alike—all those who resisted the excesses of the Counter-Reformation:

> Quand je regarde cete ardeur indomptable dequoy tant de milliers d'hommes, femmes et enfans, se presentent et rejettent à tant de fois aux dangers inevitables, pour la deffence de leurs dieux et de leur liberté; céte genereuse obstination de souffrir toutes extremitz et difficultez, et la mort, plus volontiers que de se soubmettre à la domination de ceux de qui ils ont esté si honteusement abusez. (910B/694)

> When I consider that indomitable ardor with which so many thousands of men, women, and children came forth and hurled themselves so many times into inevitable dangers for the defense of their gods and of their liberty, and that noble, stubborn readiness to suffer all extremities and hardships, even death, rather than submit to the domination of those by whom they have been so shamefully deceived.

Moral conviction inspired the Aztecs and Incas, as it did the most faithful Jews and Protestants, to follow their beliefs. The moral courage described above could be applied to those Protestants who remained inside their churches to be burned to death rather than emerging to face forced conversion. Montaigne's description of his own moral efforts to battle the onset of seasickness rather than surrender his physical body to the care of physicians brings me back to the analogy between the physical body and the body politic or spiritual congregation.

Géralde Nakam has identified the essay "De la phisionomie" as the essay to represent the final years of Henri III and the years when Montaigne was the most personally threatened by the Wars of Religion.[17] It is no coincidence that it is in this essay that one sees the most frequent analogies between the health of the individual and the health of the body politic. For six months in 1587, the essayist and his family went from town to town when the nearby town of Castillon-la-Bataille was besieged by the *Ligue* and pestilence overtook the population: "J'escriois cecy environ le temps qu'une forte charge de nos trouble se croupit plusieurs mois, de tout son pois, droict sur moy" (III: 12, 1041B/796) [I was writing this about the time when a mighty load of our disturbances settled down for several months with all its weight right on me]. Although Catholics and Protestants lived side by side in the area around Castillon-la-Bataille, Montcaret, and Ste-Foy-la-Grande, Montaigne uses a political label rather than a religious label to speak of the manner in which his neighbors viewed his allegiance:

> J'encorus les inconveniens que la moderation aporte en telles maladies. Je fus pelaudé à toutes mains: au Gibelin j'estois Guelphe, au Guelphe Gibelin. . . . La situation de ma maison et l'acointance des hommes de mon voisinage me presentoient d'un visage, ma vie et mes actions d'un autre. (III: 12, 1044B/798)

> I incurred the disadvantages that moderation brings in such maladies. I was belabored from every quarter; to the Ghibelline I was a Guelph, to the Guelph a Ghibelline. . . . The situation of my house and my acquaintance with men in my neighborhood presented me in one aspect, my life and my actions in another.

The allusion to the political parties in Florence's civil strife in lieu of the religious factions in France reveals that Montaigne is grounded in the civil threat—the loss of the body politic through the struggle between religious factions. It is here that he summons all his venom for the ills of civil strife: "En ces maladies populaires, on peut distinguer sur le commencent les sains des malades; mais quand elles viennent à durer, comme la nostre, tout le corps s'en sent, et la teste et les talons; aucune partye n'est exempte de corruption" (1042B/796) [In these epidemics one can distinguish at the beginning the well from the sick; but when they come to last, like ours, the whole body is affected, head and heels alike; no part is free from corruption]. Montaigne's description of the later stages of the disease reminds one of the various stages in the progression of syphilis, where first the pustules appear on the private parts, but later there is hair loss and excruciating pain in the joints resulting from the disease attacking the membranes covering the bones (Quétal, 57).

I spoke above of Fioravanti's tendency to dwell on the symptoms instead of on the root cause of the illness. Here, the empirical Montaigne describes the symptoms of civil war—corrupting all parts of the body politic.[18] I am reminded of Starobinski's statement that when Montaigne describes himself, he does so in medical discourse—so too for his description of the political ills that threaten the monarchy and unity of the kingdom of France. As syphilis or the plague ravages the body parts one by one, so, too, civil war and, indeed, the Wars of Religion, destroyed laws, family ties, and political allegiances. Reformation can in fact lead to deformity: "renversant la police, le magistrat et les loix en la tutelle desquelles Dieu l'a colloqué, desmembrant sa mere et en donnant à ronger les pieces à ses anciens ennemis, remplissant des haines parricides les courages fraternels" (1043C/798) [by overthrowing the government, the authorities, and the laws under whose tutelage God has placed him, by dismembering his mother and giving pieces to her ancient enemy to gnaw on, by filling the hearts of brothers with parricidal hatreds]. By the time of this essay, Montaigne sees violence and inhumanity on both sides of the struggle.

He will take instruction, he adds in a later addition to the essay, from the present troubles as he has from the ancient histories: "Je m'aggrée aucunement de veoir de mes yeux ce notable spectacle de *nostre mort publique, ses symptomes et sa forme*. Et puis que je ne la puis retarder, suis content d'estre destiné à y assister et m'en instruire" (III: 12, 1046C/800; emphasis mine) [So my curiosity makes me feel some satisfaction at seeing with my own eyes this notable spectacle of our *public death, its symptoms* and *its form*. And since I cannot retard it, I am glad to be destined to watch it and learn from it.] He is at the bedside of his moribund country and reads the symptoms in order to learn from them. His text becomes a record of the devastation of civil war for future generations, just as Dante's and Petrarch's work were for Montaigne. Called to rescue his own family from siege and pestilence, he stops writing: "Moy qui suis si hospitalier, fus en tres penible queste de retraicte pour ma famille; une famille esgarée, faisant peur à ses amis et à soy-mesme, et horreur où qu'elle cerchast à se placer, ayant à changer de demeure soudain qu'un de la troupe commençoit à se douloir au bout du doigt" (1048B/801-2) [I, who am so hospitable, had a great deal of trouble finding a retreat for my family: a family astray, a source of fear to their friends and themselves, and of horror wherever they sought to settle, having to shift their abode as soon as one of the group began to feel pain in the end of his long finger].

After the fact, once the double siege of outer threat and inner threat have passed, he takes up his written diagnostic of two illnesses: the collective one that continues to threaten the country and the individual sickness that threatens his own body—the congenital illness of kidney stones that felled his father and grandfather before him. He has grown used to the second illness, but it is the first that has moved him beyond his usual calm and focused approach: "Tout cela m'eust beaucoup moins touché si je n'eusse eu à me ressentir de la peine d'autruy, et servir six mois miserablement de guide—à cette caravane. Car je porte en moy *mes preservaifs*, qui sont *resolution et souffrance*" (III: 12, 1048B/802; emphasis mine) [All this would have affected me much less if I had not had to feel for the sufferings of others and serve for six months of misery as guide to this caravan. For I carry my own preservatives within me, which are resolution and patience].

By conflating the health of the individual and the health of the nation, the essayist suggests that in the presence of collective violence and breach of law—"la police, le magistrat et les loix"—the best recourse is resolute behavior and forbearance (III: 12, 1043B/798). His statement recalls Ronsard's comment in response to his Calvinist critics that he remains a "Tres-humble observateur des loix et de mon Prince" ("Response aux injures et calomnies," *Oeuvres complètes,* II: 606, v. 31). Montaigne's (and Ronsard's) instinct to respect the rule of law would be the internal moral rudder when the outside becomes unpredictable and at odds with established law. To show how these two "preventative remedies" work, the essayist offers the two examples from his personal life in "De la phisionomie": the attack by local partisans of the Catholic *Ligue* on Montaigne's own estate and Montaigne's temporary capture during one of his missions to Paris. In both cases, it is his outer calm and forthright behavior that save the day.

The final essay, "De l'experience," takes the reader from the public context of historic events that are laid out in "De la phisionomie" to the individual situation of Montaigne—his health, his habits, his motive for writing. As Jean Starobinski has observed, the essayist's remarks about his health take on the form of a medical questionnaire of the type one fills in when going in for a medical check-up (Starobinski, 296):

> In summary, Montaigne, beginning from his personal experience, is filling in, so to speak, the questionnaire that professional medicine formulates in general terms, and whose headings he had himself enumerated in the last essay of Book II, when he had evoked the diverse considerations of which the medical profession should keep itself informed, at the risk, otherwise, of "se mesconter" if one of these considerations is poorly grounded: "la complexion de malade, sa temperature, ses humeurs, ses inclinations, ses actions, ses pensemens mesmes et ses imaginations" [his patient's condition, his temperament, his humors, his inclinations, his actions, his very thoughts and fancies]. (II: 37, 773A/586)

Montaigne is in fact giving a experiential diagnostic not only for his own health but for the body politic. The kingdom of France relies on each person to exert his or her own moral compass in order to emerge from the sick times caused by the civil and religious strife. In "De l'experience," Montaigne comments on the sound advice of Tiberius, who might have learned the rule of self-monitoring one's own health from Socrates:

> Et le pouvoit avoir apprins de Socrates, lequel, conseillant à ses disciples, soigneusement et comme un tres principal estude, l'estude de leur santé, adjoustoit qu'il estoit malaisé qu'un homme d'entendement, prenant garde à ses exercices, à son boire et à son manger, ne discernast mieux que tout medecin ce qui luy estoit bon ou mauvais. (III: 13, 1079C/826–27)

> And he might have learned this from Socrates, who, advising his disciples, carefully and as a principal study, the study of their health, used to add that it was difficult for an intelligent man who was careful about his exercise, his drinking, and his eating, not to know better than any doctor what is good or bad for him.

When subjects fail to observe the rules that govern them, when the state fails to govern itself through the execution of established law, then the individual subject needs to look inward. This has been Montaigne's response:

> Car depuis quelques années aux courvées de la guerre, quand toute la nuict y court, comme il advient communéement, apres cinq ou six heures l'estomac me commence à troubler, avec vehemente douleur de teste, et n'arrive poinct au jour sans vomir. Comme les autres s'en vont desjeuner

je m'en vay dormir, et au partir de là aussi gay qu'au paravant. (III: 13, 1084B/831)

For in the last few years, being in the military service, when whole nights are spent on duty, as often happens, after five or six hours, I begin to be troubled by my stomach, as well as by a violent headache, and I do not last until daytime without vomiting. As the others are going off to breakfast I go off to sleep, and after that I am as gay as before.

Medical opinion, the essayist tells us, is as changeable as climate: "Elle change selon les climats et selon les Lunes, selon Farnel et selon l'Escale" (1087B/833) [It changes according to the climates and according to the moons, according to Fernel and according to L'Escale].[19] The state of health of the country cannot risk such changeability. It relies on the rule of law that will be the same for all subjects irrespective of religious belief.

The integration of knowledge or science within the individual understanding that comes through experience brings Montaigne to the position that the individual's experience of illness and, by extension, of disruptions in the health of the body politic, benefit from order and custom. He echoes Ambroise Paré in advocating that the patient or the old man not change his habits just because he is experiencing less robust health. Giving up meat or amorous thoughts just because one has entered into a period of physical weakness may only hasten the coldness and dryness that come as one approaches death. Keeping to one's habitual foods and activities may ensure that the individual retains the warmth and positive thinking that fights off approaching death. Starobinski quotes Paré in recommending warm and moist meat to ward off, however briefly, the cold dryness of death: "semble meilleur la [la vieillesse] des viandes contraires à son tempérament, sçavoir chaudes et humides, pour tousjours retarder les causes de la mort, frigité et siccité, qui la talonne de bien pres."[20] Avoiding abrupt changes in diet or activities, Paré continues, provides a certain stability to the patient or the aging citizen: "Ce n'est pas assez seulement d'avoir cogneu la quantité et qualité des viandes, mais aussi il faut entendre la *coustume* et maniere de les prendre" [It is not enough to have known the quantity and quality of meats but also one must understand the habit and manner of taking them].[21] To respect habit in sickness as in health is to follow nature "és sains, mais aussi és malades" (Paré, 29; Starobinski, 282–83). Montaigne maintains with Paré that he follows the same regimen in sickness and in health. He trusts his desires and inclinations: "Et sain et malade, je me suis volontiers laissé aller aux appetits qui me pressoient. Je donne grande authorité à mes desirs et proprensions" (III: 13, 1086B/832) [Both in health and in sickness I have readily let myself follow my urgent appetites. I give great authority to my desires and inclinations]. Restricting his diet or his activities would be akin to curing one ill by another: "Je n'ayme point à guarir le mal par le mal" (1086B/832) [I do not like to cure trouble by trouble]. Experience—whether in the sickness of an individual or the body politic—is grounded in habit, the equilibrium that custom provides. "L'experience m'a encores appris cecy, que nous nous perdons d'impatience. Les maux ont leur vie et leurs bornes, leurs maladies et leur santé" (III: 13, 1088B and C/834) [Experience has further taught me this, that we ruin ourselves by impatience. Troubles have their life and their limits, their illnesses and their health].

For the patient and for the French subject, introducing new experiments, innovations, and laws can only prolong the illness, the disturbance. Curing this "monstrueuse guerre" requires a return to the order that existed prior to the dissolution of public order. When Montaigne attributes to the Wars of Religion the capacity to self-destruct with their own venom, he calls to all French subjects to return to the rule of law: "Monstrueuse guerre: les autres agissent au dehors; cette-cy encore contre soy se ronge et se desfaict par son propre venin. Elle est de nature si maligne et ruineuse qu'elle se ruine quand et quand le reste, et se deschire et desmembre de rage" (III: 12, 1041B/796) [Monstrous war! Other wars act outward; this one acts also against itself, eats and destroys itself by its own venom. It is by nature so malignant and ruinous that it ruins itself together with all the rest and tears and dismembers itself with rage].[22] I might note Brenton Hobart's insight when he states that in most narratives of pestilence, corruption in morals follows the outbreak of the epidemic. For Montaigne, moral decay precedes the epidemic (Hobart, 403).

The language used in the description of this "monstrous war" reminds me of the violence and virulence often used to describe syphilis—which brings me back to the nexus mentioned in the title of this study: syphilis, cannibalism, and empirical medicine. Alfred W. Crosby Jr. speaks of "widespread rashes and ulcers, often extending into the mouth and throat; severe fevers and bone pains; and often early death."[23] Ulrich von Hutten, writing in 1540, vividly describes the symptoms:

> There were byles, sharpe and standing out, hauyng the similitude and quantite of Acornes, from which come so foule humours, and so great

stenche, that who so ever ones smelled it, thought hym selfe to be enfect. The colour of these pusshes [pustules] was darke grene, and the sight thereof was more grievous unto the Pacient then the peyne it selfe; and yet their peynes were as thoughe they had layn in fire."[24]

Von Hutten, one of the many correspondents of Erasmus, documents the approximate date of the appearance of the French disease in Europe: "In the yere of Chryst 1493 or there about . . . this most foule and most grevous dysease beganne to sprede."[25] Crosby notes that it was with the information that guaiac wood was effective in treating the patient suffering from syphilis that the connection was made between the discovery of the New World and the outbreak of this dreaded illness (Crosby, 220). It was a surgeon like Fioravanti, Ruis Díaz de Isla, who "claimed in a book first published in 1539 that he had treated some of Columbus's men who had contracted syphilis in 1492 in America and that he had observed its rapid spread in Barcelona" (Crosby, 222).

The chronicles, the stories of cannibalism, and the spread of a virulent new disease captivated the intellectual and scientific imagination of the Old World. Reports of empirical medical cures that grew out of the culture in which the disease originated gave rise to an emerging interest in empirical medicine. Old World science failed where New World remedies proved efficacious. Montaigne took home from his "cannibales" a perspective on the power of observation and respect for integrity of the individual (mind and body). He drew from his personal experience of illness a parallel on the well-being of the greater social order. Just as it is important for the physician not to upset the rhythm and routine of the patient, so too, moral stability strengthens the social body through long and steady observance of social laws. Montaigne understood that cannibalism was a cultural practice integrated solidly into the everyday life of the social order and represented a ritual that brought strength and stability to society. His third book of essays is a reflection on how abrupt changes in social and medical regimens disrupt and weaken the health of the individual and the well-being of the collective subjects of the kingdom. As will be evident in chapter 6, Montaigne was not alone in concluding that France suffered from a self-inflicted illness. Agrippa d'Aubigné believed that the French state was infected with an internal illness, or "maladie implicite," in which the will of one segment of society to harm the other had weakened the kingdom.[26]

6

Tragic Afflictions
D'Aubigné's Tragiques

As I have shown in previous chapters, the virulence and rapid spread of syphilis in Europe in the first half of the sixteenth century provided a metaphor for the violence and chaos caused by the French Wars of Religion. How else to explain the language of festering sores to describe heresy ("Une heresie puante / est fluante") in the manner of Artus Désiré or Montaigne's manner of characterizing the period of the Wars of Religion as "our public death, with its symptoms and form" ("Nostre mort publique, ses symptomes et sa forme")?[1] The spiritual sickness brought on by the civil strife between Catholics and Protestants provoked a physical breakdown visible in the disruption in family ties, the failure of princes to look after the well-being of all their citizens, and the corruption of legal practices. Acts of peace—what might be viewed as remedies—glossed over old sores. As a consequence, civil strife went into remission, only to recur in a more violent form, much as the mercury treatments for syphilis later caused insufferable pain in the joints and gradually poisoned the entire body.[2] Jeff Persels has noted that the twentieth and twenty-first centuries are not alone in resorting to the "figurative potential of mortal infirmity." "Venereal disease (syphilis, gonorrhea) and melancholia are but two of the most familiar 'maux du siècle' of the sixteenth century."[3]

Andrea Frisch has described the importance of witnessing for Huguenots. It is through the mediation of the Holy Spirit that the believing Christian feels the symbolic meaning of the holy Eucharist, as represented by the bread and the wine: "The Holy Spirit in Calvin's theology is the paradigmatic symbol of efficacious—yet (or, from the Protestant point of view *because*) transparent—testimony of one world [human] to another [divine]."[4] D'Aubigné establishes himself from the beginning of *Les Tragiques* as an eyewitness to the disturbing violence that forces Mother France to choose between her two children—Catholics ("cet Esau") and Protestants ("son Jacob")—those who seek to persecute and those who uphold the liberty of conscience:[5] "Car mes yeux sont tesmoings du subjet de mes vers" ("Misères," *Les Tragiques*, 284, v. 371). Yet he enlists the help of his compatriots: "Vous n'estes spectateurs, vous estes personages" ("Misères," *Les Tragiques*, 272, v. 170). To have seen is to take an active part in witnessing the violence. It is the collective suffering—the blow to what had been a united people—that lies at the heart of his work. Every French person was an actor in the tragedy and was pulled willingly or unwillingly into harm's way.

Jean-Raymond Fanlo is clear in his assessment that *Les Tragiques*, in spite of some passages composed in the era of Henri III, is not a work dictated at the time of the events and in the heat of the violence: "Ils n'ont pas jailli 'au milieu des armees,' ils ont été composés dans un cabinet de travail livres en main" (*Les Tragiques*, I: 117) [They didn't spring up in the midst of armies, they were composed books in hand in a study]. Fanlo points out that it is not only the books that surround d'Aubigné in his study, but memories—here understood as both memoirs and reminiscences—his own reflections and those penned by others:

> Mais il faut aussi, compte tenu du laps de temps écoulé entre l'événement et sa formulation poétique, considérer le métier sur lequel l'oeuvre a été tissée, ainsi que les enjeux nouveaux de cette rhétorique passionnée mise en oeuvre dans un cabinet de travil en province, au milieu de livres et de mémoires. (*Les Tragiques*, I: 117; translation mine)

> But we need also, considering the lapse of time between the event and its poetic formulation, consider the loom on which the work was woven, as well as the innovative stakes for this fervent rhetoric carried out in the provincial study amidst books and memoirs.

The whole work, or *oeuvre,* as opposed to brief passages that may date from an earlier period, is clearly the product of what Dominick LaCapra calls secondary memory. It is not the immediate work of memory as a lived experience, with its "lapses relating to denial, repression, suppression, and evasion," but the result of secondary memory on those earlier experiences "that leads to the emergence of both a more accurate memory and a clearer appraisal of what is or is not factual remembrance."[6] D'Aubigné has had the time to process the suffering and violence and, now as "participant" and "observer," along with his compatriots—Protestants or Catholics—"they may conceivably agree on certain things that constitute accurate memory. They may even debate the relevance of that memory for social and political life in the present and the future" (LaCapra, 21). It is the passage of time—the thoughtful work in the "cabinet de travail"—that provides the continuity, the staying power of d'Aubigné's narration and rhetoric.

D'Aubigné was not alone in postponing the composition of his account of the violent circumstances of the French Wars of Religion. Like Jean de Léry, who would wait almost twenty years to publish his *Histoire d'un voyage faict en la terre du Brésil*, or Montaigne, whose traumatic experience fleeing an outbreak of the plague and the civil unrest in his immediate region interrupted his writing of the *Essais*, d'Aubigné waited to reconstruct "from its effects and traces" the events he recounts so vividly (LaCapra, 21). Montaigne, forced to leave home and to take his wife and daughter on the road, broke off his writing: "Moy qui suis si hospitalier, fus en tres penible queste de retraicte pour ma famille: une famille esgarée faisant peur à ses amis et à soy-mesme" (*Les Essais,* III: 12, 1048B/801–02) [I, who am so hospitable, had a great deal of trouble finding a retreat for my family: a family astray, a source of fear to their friends and themselves]. Words such as *esgarée* and *peur* attest to the trauma of the event, which during the direct experience prevented being "integrated into experience or directly remembered" (LaCapra, 21).[7] Through secondary memory, the writer will come back to the experience to commit it to more articulate and coherent narration. Such is d'Aubigné's approach to *Les Tragiques*.

A notable exception to this lapse of time between witnessing a traumatic or troubling event and writing about it is Léry's *Histoire mémorable du siège de Sancerre* (1573), an account that has significant echoes in d'Aubigné's narration of starvation and suffering undergone by the Huguenots. As Léry explains, the leader of the siege on the largely but not exclusively Protestant inhabitants of Sancerre, Claude de La Châtre, requests that Léry, one of the besieged, create an account of how the besieged managed to hold out for so long against the royal forces.

Because of his experience with battling hunger and yet surviving on the return journey from Brazil, Léry was thought to have instructed his fellow Huguenots at Sancerre on survival tactics and thus to have prolonged their resistance. Léry replies humbly to La Châtre that it was the ingenuity ("invention") of those of his religion and not his experience that accounted for the long resistance. In this case, it was indeed necessity being the mother of invention ("la necessité maistresse des arts"). La Châtre requests a "discours de la famine."[8] Just prior to unleashing his anger at seeing the town razed by the royal forces and writing in all capital letters "ICY FUT SANCERRE," Léry presents his account to La Châtre ("le discours de nostre famine"; 335). He claims his part in the suffering with the possessive pronoun *nostre*. D'Aubigné would have no better model in painting what Géralde Nakam calls the "phénomène de la faim" than Jean de Léry (*Au lendemain de la Saint-Barthélemy*, 100). That hunger is front and center in Les Tragiques is clear early on in "Misères," where the eyewitness narrator states: "Là de mille maisons, on ne trouva que feux, / Que charognes, que morts, ou visages affreux: / La faim va devant moi, force est que je la suive: / J'oy d'un gosier mourant une voix demi-vive" (*Les Tragiques*, I: 284, vv. 379–82) [There of a thousand houses, we find only fires, / only carcasses, only dead bodies or frightful faces / Hunger goes in front of me, I feel constrained to follow it: / From a dying throat comes a half-dead voice].

Painting physical and moral suffering lies at the heart of d'Aubigné's work: "Je veux peindre la France une mere affligee" ("Misères," *Les Tragiques*, I: 267, v. 97). Mother France is depicted as the afflicted mother, witness to her two sons fighting over her breasts for milk, an allegory mentioned by Frank Lestringant (*Une sainte horreur*, 67). While Esau, representing the Catholics, is the instigator, wasting the sweet milk that ought to be enough to feed two ("faict degast de doux laict, qui doibt nourir les deux"; "Misères," *Les Tragiques*, I: 268, v. 104), his brother Jacob, a veiled symbol of the Protestants, defends himself with good reason against the aggression of the brother, but the field of battle is their mother's body ("dont le champ est la mere"; "Misères," *Les Tragiques*, I: 268, v. 110). In spite of acting in self-defense, Jacob, along with his aggressive bother Esau, is accused by Mother France of being mutinous ("mutins"; 269, v. 119) and felonious ("felons"; 269, v. 127) for having bloodied the breast that nourished them: "Elle dit, vous avez felons ensanglanté / Le sein qui vous nourrit" (269, vv. 127–28).

D'Aubigné transforms "Mother France" into a disease-ridden body whose humoral balance is destroyed, producing a state of dyscrasia, a state in which the black bile caused by melancholy is deposited in the liver (*Les Tragiques*, I: 271, n. 145–46):

> Ce vieil corps tout infect plein de sa discratie
> Hydropique faict l'eau, si bien que ce geant
> Qui alloit de ses nerfs ses voisins outrageant
> ("Misères," *Les Tragiques*, I: 271, vv. 146–48)

> This old body all infected full of discrasia
> Dropsied produces water, so that this giant
> Proceeds through its strength to harm its neighbors

The swelling that results from dropsy (*hydropie*) keeps the stomach from processing ingested food ("N'envoye plus aux bords les justes aliments"; 271, v 152) and from nourishing the organs, leaving the legs and arms without essential marrow ("Des jambes et des bras les os sont sans moëlle"; 271, v. 153).[9] The brain is poisoned by improperly filtered fluids (271, vv. 154–55). The swollen body renders the legs unable to support its weight ("Les jambes sans pouvoir porter leur masse lourde"; 271, v. 161).

The intensely detailed physical description of France's infected body doubles as a moral and political description of the gradual starving of the populace. The people, the belly of France, or "Vous ventre de la France, enflé de vos langueurs" (272, v. 167) [You belly of France swollen in your weakened state], are described as victims of dropsy, swollen, starved by the schism that sets brother against brother in a kind of suicide (*autochyre*; v. 189). The stronger suffers at least as much as the weaker, for what was once whole and unified is lost (273, vv. 189–90).

Like Léry, d'Aubigné becomes witness to the starvation inflicted on the peasants by the German mercenaries, recruited, as Fanlo notes, by Huguenots and Catholics alike ("Misères," *Les Tragiques*, I: 284, n. 372).[10] D'Aubigné states: "Car mes yeux sont tesmoings du subject de mes vers" [284, v. 371] [For my eyes are witness to the subject of my verses]. He evokes the voice of a Perigordin, that "half-dead voice" mentioned earlier, bearing testimony to the cannibalism of the mercenaries as he beseeches his compatriots to kill him to put an end to further suffering:

> Faictes-moy d'un bon coup, et promptement mourir,
> Les reistres m'ont tué par faute de viande,
> D'un coup de coutelas, l'un d'eux m'a emporté
> . . . .

Ce bras que vous voyez pres du lict à costé:
("Misères," *Les Tragiques*, I: 285, vv. 392–96)

Hit me with a solid blow, so that I die promptly,
The mercenaries killed me since they had no meat
With a blow of the cutlass, one of them dispatched
. . . .
This arm that you see near the bed just beside:

As Léry had done before him, d'Aubigné remarks upon the dismembered limb as proof of the cannibalistic intentions of the mercenaries.[11] As if to parallel the image of the dropsied "Mother France," d'Aubigné paints "l'horrible anathomie / De la mere assechee" ("Misères," *Les Tragiques*, I: 286, vv. 414–15) [the ghastly anatomy of the dried up mother] who in vain tries to rescue her children. Here the reader notes, as Lestringant suggests, the image of the martyred child or "l'enfant martyr," pure inside but bloodied outside by the acts of the vicious papists (*Une sainte horreur*, 81). The child is the opposite of the communion host as understood by the Catholics, which is white on the outside, but through the act of transubstantiation, becomes red inside as it is transformed into the real body of Jesus Christ: "L'Eucharistie catholique enveloppe l'enfant Jésus de pâte et déguise le crime alimentaire sous l'apparence anodin du pain" (*Une sainte horreur*, 81) [The Catholic host wraps up the baby Jesus in pastry and disguises the dietary crime with the harmless appearance of bread].

The distraught voice of the hapless eyewitness from Périgord invites one to witness, if one has the stomach for more suffering ("Helas! si vous avez encore quelque envie / De voir plus de mal-heur"; 286, vv. 406–7), the demise of his children, but only one child remains, the other presumably consumed by the soldiers in lieu of suitable meat. The portrait of the blood spilling over the child from the mother's mortal wounds instead of milk from her breasts parallels Mother France's statement that she has henceforth only blood to offer her children, as a result of their fighting over her breasts to suckle. In both cases, those of Esau and Jacob and of the mercenaries, the fault lies in their disordered appetites. The severed arm of the father and the missing body of the child bear testimony to the starvation and suffering caused by internal civil strife. France as they know it is dying, "ce corps seché, retraict, / De la France qui meurt fut un autre pourtraict" (*Les Tragiques*, 286, 423–24) [this dry, shriveled up body / Was another portrait of the dying France]. In a testimony of cruel persecution, there must be evidence of "wild appetites" that stretch well beyond the rules governing the normal social behavior of human beings.[12] The cannibalism practiced by the mercenary soldiers in war-torn France and on a regular basis in the Catholic Mass is set in stark contrast to the innocent child martyr.

Earlier in the poem, the author has denounced the false laws that have destroyed what was once France:

> Barbares en effect, françois de nom, François,
> Vos fausses loix ont fait des faux et jeunes roys,
> Impuissants sur leurs coeurs, cruels en leur puissance:
> ("Misères," *Les Tragiques,* I: 273, vv. 191–93)

> Barbarous in fact, French by name, French,
> Your unjust laws have created unjust and young kings,
> Weak in controlling their bodies, cruel in their power:

D'Aubigné, as Montaigne had done, blames the civil unrest on the failure to follow the laws of the land—the principles that guide consistent human interaction. Laws protect the individual from his or her own inconsistencies, Montagine observes: "Les loix m'ont osté de grand peine; elles m'ont choisy party et donné un maistre" (*Les Essais,* III: 1, 794–95B/603) [The laws have freed me from great anxiety; they have chosen me my party and given me a master]. Géralde Nakam has commented on the tension in "De la phisionomie" between the violence of the eighth religious war and Montaigne's anger at the suffering it caused the people.[13] The essayist, as does d'Aubigné, remarks on the importance of discipline, discipline that comes not from foreign mercenaries but from the French army: "Nos armées ne se lient et tiennent plus que par simant estranger: des françois on ne sçait plus faire le corps d'armée constant et reglé" (*Les Essais,* III: 12, 1042B/796) [Our arms are no longer bound and held together except by foreign cement; of Frenchmen on can no longer form a steadfast and disciplined army corps]. He adds that "il n'y a qu'autant de discipline que nous en font voir des soldats empruntez; quant à nous, nous nous conduisons à discretion, et non pas de chef, chacun selon la sienne" (III: 12, 1042B/796) [there is only so much discipline as borrowed soldiers show us; as for ourselves, we follow our own lead and not our leader's, every man in his own way].

D'Aubigné shows where these borrowed customs lead—to an absence of self-control and respect for French laws and customs that restrain the behavior of kings and peasants. Chaos results from kings giving up their role as upholders of the law. They become "ravisseurs de pucelles; / Adulteres souillans les couches des plus belles" ("Misères," *Les Tragiques*, I: 274, vv. 201–2) [violators of maidens; / Adulterers soiling the beds of the most beautiful women]. D'Aubigné goes beyond Léry in depicting the moral confusion that compels a mother to choose between love of her child and the gnawing hunger that makes her forget her maternal instinct to protect her child from harm. Hunger snatches the title of mother from the starving woman and replaces her with a famished being:

> La mere ayant long-temps combatu dans son coeur,
> Le feu de la pitié, de la faim la fureur,
> Convoitte dans son sein la creature aimee,
> Et dit à son enfant (moins mere qu'affamee)
> Rend miserable, rends le corps que je t'ay faict:
> Ton sang retournera, où tu as pris le laict,
> Au sein qui t'allaictoit r'entre contre nature,
> Ce sein qui t'a nourry sera ta sepulture.
> ("Misères," *Les Tragiques*, I: 291, vv. 519–26)

> The mother having long fought in her heart
> The fire of pity and the furor of hunger,
> Covets in her breast this beloved creature
> And says to her child as less mother than starving woman
> Give over wretched child, give over the body that I made for you;
> Your blood will return to where you suckled
> To the breast which nursed you return against all rules of nature,
> This breast which suckled you will be your tomb.

The act of infanticide for the sake of nourishing herself and perhaps others is a struggle. Her reluctant hand drops the knife twice ("Deux fois le fer eschappe à la main qui roidit"; *Les Tragiques*, I: 291, v. 532), yet hunger wins out over maternal love as she, instead of kissing the child, tears the flesh of the child with her teeth: "Elle n'appreste plus les levres, mais les dents, / Et des baisers changez en avides blessures"; 291, vv. 536–37).[14] What has brought this transgression of custom, faith, and law to pass? Conscience is outwitted by both hunger and reason ("la faim et la raison / Donnent pasture au corps, et à l'ame poison," ["Misères," *Les Tragiques*, I: 292, vv. 559–60] [hunger and reason / Feed the body and poison the soul]). It is the mother who will pay with her soul for having transgressed her responsibilities as mother, yet d'Aubigné condemns the tyrannical influence of the *Ligue* on the throne of France, and demands a return to a benevolent monarchy in which the monarchs took seriously their responsibilities as "vrais peres et vrais rois" [true fathers and true kings] to feed their people as "Nourrissons de la France" [Providers of France]. The civil wars, where both Henri III and Henri de Navarre fought against the tyranny and intolerance of the *Ligue* and the Guise family, have caused the suffering.[15] The *Ligue*, as the unknown murderer ("meurtrier inconnu"), is indeed judged guilty ("coulpable tenu"; "Misères," *Les Tragiques*, I: 293, vv. 591–92). The people facing the starvation and violence are hard put to discern by which party the cruel mercenaries have been sent. And it is for this reason that Montaigne clings to the law as his choice of party—it is more consistent and relieves him of choosing allegiance (passage previously cited; III: I, 794–95B/603). But it is clear to for the author of the *Tragiques*, who lays the blame for dividing the people of France and tormenting them on "une fatale femme, un cardinal qui d'elle, / Parangon de malheur, suivoit l'ame cruelle" ("Misères," *Les Tragiques*, 301, vv. 725–26) [a fatal woman, a cardinal who / follows her cruel soul, paragon of evil].

As the Huguenot Léry had done, d'Aubigné attributes the unnatural acts of cannibalism and the corrupted morals of the people to France's pride in turning to superstitions ("superstitions"), corrupted habits ("coustume folles"), and idols ("idolles"), here described as foreign evils ("maux estrangers").[16] Instead of turning to God ("Ce grand Dieu void au ciel du feu de son clair oeil" ["Misères," *Les Tragiques*, I: 298, vv. 687] [This great God sees in heaven with the fire of his omniscient eye]), France has given way to pride, and the peace contracted was only the bastard sister of peace; nothing was honored but vice ("Ta paix estoit la soeur bastarde de la paix: / Rien n'estoit honoré parmy toy que le vice"; "Misères," *Les Tragiques*, I: 299, vv. 692–93). Catherine de Medici had led the rival factions of France's religious and civil wars to turn against the county's best interests: "Et un peuple par toy contre soy mutiné" ("Misères," *Les Tragiques*, 304, v. 776).

In "Misères," Catherine de Medici is seconded by the powerful Cardinal de Lorraine, painted by d'Aubigné in the cardinal red, a scarlet reflecting not only the victims of persecution but also his libidinous character ("paillardise"): a licentious individual, sodomite, and incestuous defiler of the bed of his sister-in-law Anne d'Este ("adultere, paillard, bougre, et incestueux"; 316, v. 1004).[17] His death, in Avignon in December 1574, described in "Vengeances," Book VI of *Les Tragiques*, was accompanied by a violent storm signaling the death of so many devils ("tant de diables moururent"; 851, v. 1038). Again, corrupt morals, unhealthy sexual acts, are at the root of France's schism. Recall that in Léry's work, *Histoire d'un voyage faict en la terre du Brésil,* "paillardise" is linked both to the description of the sexuality of the cannibals in the New World and to the corrupt and godless Norman interpreters of the Tupi language and culture ("où vivans sans crainte de de Dieu, ils paillardoyent avec les femmes et filles" [180/43] [where, having no fear of God, they lived in wantonness with women and girls]).[18] For d'Aubigné, the Cardinal de Lorraine's wanton private life is juxtaposed to the corrupt régime of the judges who carry out his orders and those of the Queen Mother:

> Nous avons parmy nous cette gent cannibale
> ....
> ... et de leurs mains fumantes
> Portent à leur palais bras et mains innocentes,
> Font leur chair de la chair des orphelins occis:
> ("La Chambre dorée," *Les Tragiques,* I: 443, vv. 197–203)
>
> We have among us a cannibalistic people
> ....
> ... and with their steaming hands
> Bring to their palates [mouths] innocent arms and hands,
> Consuming the flesh of slaughtered orphans:

As in the case of the Norman interpreters, the judges have abandoned reasoned justice for graft, law for force ("par dons non par raison," "la force et non le droict"; "La Chambre dorée," *Les Tragiques,* I: 445, vv. 235–36). "L'injustice impudente" has corrupted the law and risks destroying the true Church. D'Aubigné makes an appeal to the Lord to intervene to save the Church: "Vien, Seigneur, et te haste: / Car l'homme de peché, ton Eglise degaste: / Vien, dict l'esprit, accours, pour deffendre le tien: / Vien, dict l'espouse, et nous avec l'espouse, vien" ("La Chambre dorée," *Les Tragiques,* I: 498, vv. 1059–62) [Come, Lord, and hurry: / For sinful man is ruining your Church / Comme, says the spirit, run to defend what is yours; / Come, says the spouse, and we utter with the spouse, come].

Vice is not the purview only of the Queen Mother nor of the Cardinal de Lorraine, but of the royal offspring as well. Henri III is described as "degenere Henry" and the narrator alludes to "l'ordure de tes nuicts" ("Princes," *Les Tragiques,* I: 401–2, vv. 985, 994) [your filthy nights]. The rumored clandestine births of Marguerite de Valois's illegitimate baby and those of her ladies in waiting are also evoked: "Les filles de la cour sont galantes honnestes, / Qui se font bien servir, moins chastes, plus secrettes, / Qui sçavent le mieux feindre un mal pour accoucher" ("Princes," 403, vv. 1019–21; see also 403, n. 1027–35) [The young ladies of the court are gallant, honest / Who are well served less chaste and more secret / Who know how to feign sickness in order to give birth [in secret]]. Having criticized their effeminate clothing and gaudy makeup, the narrator weighs the vice of remaining silent or the virtue of bringing such corrupted mores to light.[19] Virtue's task is to uncover the infection and its festering smell: "Mieux vaut à descouvert monstrer l'infection / Avec sa puanteur, et sa punition" ("Princes," *Les Tragiques*, I: 409, 1093–94) [Better to bring to light the infection / with its festering smell and punishment]. He evokes Saint Augustine ("Le bon pere affriquain"; 409, 1095) in explaining why he is exposing the degenerate morals of the royal family. The horror of his writing leads him to drop the pen, and his tears wet his parchment: "Icy je vay laver ces papiers de mes larmes"; 409, 1103).

In a world where tyranny and persecution had driven French people to starve their brothers and sisters and to transgress the most basic of laws, death and release to a higher realm was preferable to life ruled by unnatural acts: wanton sexuality and the willful imposition of starvation on one's own compatriots, an act that led to cannibalism. D'Aubigné describes the soul looking down from above on the diseased body: "L'ame, des yeux du ciel, voit au ciel l'invisible, / Le mal horrible au corps, ne luy est pas horrible" ("Les Fers," *Les Tragiques*, I: 545, vv. 857–58) [The soul, with heaven's eyes, sees the invisible in heaven, the hideous diseased body does not instill fear]. The many inhumane torture devices devised by human beings are releases for those who scorn death: "qui mesprise la mort, que luy fera de tort / Le regard asseuré des outils de la mort?" (545, vv. 855–56) [To someone who scorns death, what harm can come from / The reassuring look of instruments of death?].

Facing death nobly, choosing union with God rather than a life that obeys no laws, human, natural, or divine, the exemplary martyrs d'Aubigné describes have learned the art of dying well. Bound to a post and awaiting death, Estienne Brun asks his son: "N'as-tu peu bien vivant apprendre à bien mourir?" ("Les Feux," *Les Tragiques*, I: 548, b. 932) [Haven't you been able to learn to die well while living well?]. Choosing reunion with her Savior in preference to life in a world where innocent children are tortured, one of the daughters of Minister Serpon, tortured and bleeding, raises her bloodied hand to implore God to take her to him in death as she has lived in and through him in life: "Et que je meure en toy, comme en toy j'ay vescu" ("Les Feux," *Les Tragiques,* I: 553, v. 1075).[20] Catholic guards and priests, having tried to seduce her with "ordures" (here one may read Catholic doctrine and propaganda), end by cruelly withholding daily bread: "Pour dernier instrument, ils osterent le pain" (552, v. 1055). It is here that d'Aubigné cries out against the inhumanity and lawlessness of his countrymen: "O François, desreiglez, où logent voz polices/Puisque vos hospitaux servent à tels offices?" (554, vv. 1093–94). The institutions traditionally run by the religious orders to assist their countrymen have become instruments of torture—the same "outils de la mort" mentioned earlier.

Finally, the bestial nature of the persecution is revealed. In Auxerre, the dogs refuse to eat the heart and intestines of the persecuted, but the perpetrating crowd sympathetic to the Catholic cause shows no such restraint as they roast and eat the organs, savoring and swallowing the pieces like organ meat in the market. Pure appetite, unmindful of barriers to consuming the flesh of one's species, drives them on:

> Ceux-là veulent offrir leurs bergers aux mastins,
> Mais les chiens respectans le coeur et les entrailles:
> Furent comme chrestiens punis par ces canailles,
> Qui en plusieurs endroicts ont rosty, et masché,
> Savouré, avallé, tels coeurs en plain marché:
> Si quelqu'un refusoit, c'estoit à son dommage
> Qu'il n'estoit pas bien né pour estre antropophage.
> ("Les Fers," *Les Tragiques,* I: 608–9, vv. 680–86)

> Those people wanted to offer their shepherds to the mastiffs,
> But the dogs respecting the heart and the entrails,
> Were like Christians punished by the rowdy crowd,
> Who in many places roasted and chewed,
> Savored and swallowed, as one would organ meat at the market.
> If someone refused, it was at his own peril,
> That he was not born to be a cannibal.

One is at once reminded of other persecutions, such as where Jews who refused to eat pork were selected and burned at the stake, and also of the Huguenot interpretation of the Catholic theory of transubstantiation, where eating the "body of Christ" or drinking the "blood of Christ" was compared in Protestant pamphlets to cannibalism. Those who refused to savor the human flesh with the crowd remained consistent with their internal principle that consuming one's own kind was a bestial and unnatural act, forbidden by society and religion. Yet they did so at their own peril; not being born cannibals marked them as heretics.

As has been seen with Léry, cannibalism goes against all laws of nature. Fioravanti "claimed" to have experimented with pigs, dogs, and sparrow hawks. In general, they would not eat the flesh of their own kind, but if fed the flesh of their kind mixed in with other meats, they came down with the ulcers or "postules" of syphilis (Eamon, 11). The martyrs of the Reform scorn a life where wanton behavior ("paillardise") represented both in acts of cannibalism and indiscriminate sexuality, whether rape, adultery, or incest, replace the steadfast and disciplined order of an army overseen by a just head of state. The foreign mercenaries show no respect for order and Christian principles. The complete disregard for social and religious laws can have only one result—the downfall of humankind, as evidenced in the suffering brought on as a direct result of "paillardise."

It is useful to consult two documents from d'Aubigné's political writings: one to the Queen Mother, *Lettre à la Reine,* addressed to Marie de Medici, and the second, *Instruction d'Estat,* addressed to the young Duke of Montmorency, Henri II.[21] Both were written, according to Jean-Raymond Fanlo, after the coronation of the child Louis XIII, so between October 10, 1610, and the end of the year, or approximately corresponding to the final period of composition of the *Tragiques*. The author of the *Tragiques* sees a role that the Queen Mother and the young duke can play in healing the country. Not the polemical tone of the *Tragiques,* but a brief note of hope prevails in the two documents and reflects what Fanlo describes as a period of weakened royal power (*Oeuvres,* II: 184). Of interest to this study in the two documents is the sustained use of the metaphor of an ailing France in search of a cure after the violence of the Wars of Religion.

To the young *duc de Montmorency,* d'Aubigné depicts the perils of the present moment. The Queen Mother must avoid giving in to those who were most severe and unjust to the followers of Henri de Navarre before his elevation to Henri IV and to those who, pushed by ambition, seek only to flourish in the court of Louis XIII. These two factions will only harm Marie de Medici and the king, and, as d'Aubigné maintains, the kingdom is sick from subverting everything: "Le royaume est malade pour la subversion de toutes choses" (*Oeuvres,* II: 230). The duke should work to help restore the kingdom to good health by maintaining peace: "La manutention du royaume pour sa guarison, par l'entretien de sa paix" (230).

This can only be done by avoiding the two factions mentioned above and by sifting through those leaders who have suffered unjustly to choose those who will work to create a single voice ("pour faire une voix de plusieurs voix"; 231), to reduce all desires to a single wish ("tous les desirs en un desir"), different goals to a single goal ("les divers buts en un but principal"), and all the forces to a single fealty ("toutes les forces en une obeissance"; 230). D'Aubigné's image of the ideal state, ruled by one wish, one goal, and one fealty, recalls his contrast of a weakened France with celestial harmony. In the world, "les amours d'icy bas n'estoient rien que haïr" [Profane sentiments in this world below are nothing but feelings of hatred].

> Les amours d'icy bas n'estoient rien que haïr
> Au prix de hauts amours dont la saincte armonie
> Rend une ame de tous en un vouloir unie:
> Tous noz parfaicts amours reduicts en un amour
> Comme noz plus beaux jours reduicts en un beau jour
> ("Jugement," *Les Tragiques*, II: 934, vv. 1102–6)

> Profane sentiments in the world below consist only of hatred
> Compared to the lofty loves whose blessed harmony
> Transforms the soul of all into a single desire
> All our perfect loves reduced to a single love
> As our most beautiful days are reduced to a single day.

D'Aubigné gives the young duke advice for trying to achieve the difficult goal of restoring France to the order and health it had known before the chaos of the Wars of Religion, during which factionalism split a previously united spirit and vision.

D'Aubigné humbly reminds the Queen Mother that it was an unjust tyranny that had weakened France. He bids her to make her princes happy so they won't oppress the people, the officers so they won't engage in infighting, the clergy so they won't complain elsewhere (to Rome, Spain, and other Catholic allies): "Contenter vos princes sans l'oppression du peuple, voz officiers sans qu'ilz s'entrechoquent, l'ecclesiastique sans qu'il face plainte ailleurs" (*Oeuvres*, II: 195). D'Aubigné then explains himself further. He calls the French state afflicted with an internal illness, where one person's remedy infects another with ulcerous sores: "Voylà pourquoy j'appeloys les maladies de cet estat implicites quand le remede de l'un ulcere l'autre" (196). He seeks a common remedy that restores both sides to good health. What is needed is to enter the sick room ("entrer dans la chambre") with a vial of medicine ("avec la fiole à la main"). The remedy is a potion as unpleasant and bitter as rhubarb to the lips and palate ("le nom en desplaist comme celuy de la rubarbe, ce n'est qu'amertume aux levres & palais"). Yet, it contains life, joy, and perfect health within ("c'est vie, santé, joye et parfaite guerizon au dedans"; *Oeuvres*, II: 196).

Before he begins his prescription for how to restore France to good health, he expresses skepticism about the patient: "Mais peut estre ay-je plus mauvaise opinion du patient que je ne devois" (196) [Maybe I have a worse opinion of the sick person than I ought to]. There follows his advice for restoring the faith and obedience of the people, calling for the Estates-General to deliberate seriously, freely maintaining the current privileges, including the freedom of conscience to worship. In a final entreaty to the Queen Mother, he appeals to her aversion to novelty and to her fealty to the king so that she may gain the hearts of her subjects as well as their heads ("Voyla le moyen de reigner sur les coeurs ainsy que sur les testes"; 200). By reigning with a wand and not a sword, with ceremony and not force, the young king will restore his people to good health, curing the sores through peace and harmony.

With these two letters, d'Aubigné seizes a teachable moment in what Fanlo calls "une période d'affaiblissement du pouvoir royal" (Fanlo, *Écrits politiques*, II: 184), a time when royal power was weakened by the death of Henri IV and the transition to the new monarch, a young child overseen by his mother (Fanlo, *Écrits politiques*, II: 184). D'Aubigné's words to the Queen Mother and to the young Duke of Montmorency reflect the wisdom achieved through reflection on more than a half century of religious and civil disorder. It was a brief window in the long illness and what Montaigne referred to as "nostre mort publique" mentioned at the outset of this chapter. Yet, as the monarchy of Louis XIII grew stronger, and the voice of the majority grew louder, it fell to works like *Les Tragiques* and other testimonials by Huguenot pamphleteers, poets, and historians to remind the French people that a country wracked by chaos, starvation, torture, and disregard for the law is too weak to withstand external and internal threats. The leaders would need to convert spectators in the civil struggle to engaged actors in order to restore the kingdom of France to a healthy state. The unanimity of desire, goal, and fealty outlined in the *Ecrits politiques* seems to be a reflection of a heavenly ideal, found only, as it is in the last words of *Les Tragiques*, "au giron de son Dieu" [in God's bosom], rather than a realistic political solution in a France whose open sores are still festering ("Jugement," *Les Tragiques*, v. 218).

CONCLUSION

NEW DISEASES and new pandemics occasion the creation of new metaphors. In this book, I have followed just how the rapid and unexpected spread of syphilis took hold of the imagination of Renaissance thinkers and writers. The panic with which the populace confronted the disease obliges the historian, chronicler, or artist who records its onset to find a constructive rhetorical style with which to present the disease. Herein lies the importance of the metaphor, which "does not *image* the thing it seeks to characterize, *it gives directions* for finding the set of images that are intended to be associated with the thing" (White, 91). The medical treatises of the epoch, written by learned doctors and more practical surgeons, in addition to the chronicles coming back from the New World, fed the artistic output of writers composing their works as the religious controversies of the early modern period took hold and gave way to violent conflict across France and Europe. Fascination and then horror at the alarming rate at which the disease spread in the first half of the sixteenth century, along with the confirmation in such works as those of Thevet and Léry that the origins came from the wanton sexual mores of the man-eating indigenous peoples of the New World, inspired the transformation of the physical phenomenon of the disease to its embodiment as a metaphor for the spread of new religious practices.

Recall Jeff Persels' observation, mentioned in chapter 3: "Given that this current age so often has recourse to metaphors of illness . . . , we should not be . . . surprised to find earlier ages equally devoted to the figurative potential of mortal infirmity" (Persels, 1089).

The scathing rhetoric of the Catholic poet Artus Désiré, described by Jacques Pineaux as polemicizing relentlessly against the Huguenots, portrays the advance of the filthy infection of Reformist heresy as attacking the joints and weakening their appendages:[1]

> Toutes leurs Cuisses et Aynes
> Sont tant pleines
> D'heresie et de poison,
> Qui si tresfort les desgoutte
> Qu'ilz n'ont goutte
> D'apparence d'oraison,
> Eux qui souloient estre habiles
> Sont debiles
> Et leurs membres tous polus:
> Car leur orde paillardise
> Les deguise
> Tant qu'ilz en sont tout perclus.
> (Désiré, Chanson XXVI, 40)

> All their thighs and groin
> Are so full
> Of heresy and poison,
> So strongly disgusting them
> That they scarcely
> Seem to pray.
> They who used to be agile
> Are weak
> And their members so polluted:
> For their lechery
> Adulterates them
> So much that they are completely lame.

The pains and weakness in the joints, which here Désiré attributes to the heresy spread to those who were open to Calvinist preaching, are described by the surgeon Ambroise Paré as later symptoms of syphilis: "douleurs nocturnes extremes à la teste, espaules, iointures."[2] The Protestants were no less cutting in their attacks as they described the lost nose of Pierre Lizet, the former president of the parlement de Paris, as a result of syphilis: "nez boutonné / Prest à tomber par fortune / De la verole importune."[3]

The virulence of the rhetoric, like the epidemic itself, increased incrementally. As was previously noted, Rabelais and Erasmus use satire to illustrate the dangers syphilis and wanton sexuality can bring to the integrity of family living. Deaths from syphilis, combined with the behavior of lustful clerics who meddle in the affairs of the family, risk causing a decrease in the population and threaten family harmony. As the violence against the Protestants increased, so did the virulence of the rhetoric. Remember that the strident tenor of the verbal attacks on both sides occasioned in 1563 a brief halt to the inflammatory texts between Catholics and Huguenots through the Edict of September (Langer, 344). The tensions between Catholics and Protestants in France and more broadly in Europe spread to the explorers, chroniclers, and missionaries in the New World. It is at this point that the accusations of lechery and cannibalism against the indigenous populations in the New World came back to the Old World to be applied to Protestants and Catholics alike.

If the pandemic had decimated the population in Europe, the violence of the conflict between and among French countrymen and women continued the slaughter, and the people and its institutions suffered both physically and spiritually. Montaigne depicts the fraying of the moral fiber of France and the harm done to the civil institutions that are charged with maintaining order. This is indeed the "notable spectacle de nostre mort publique, ses symptomes et sa forme," to which he refers in his third book of *Essais* (III: 12, 1046C). He holds his countrymen responsible for relying on mercenaries instead of the disciplined forces that had once served the country so well. "Nos armées ne se lient et tiennent plus que par simant estranger; des françois on ne sçait plus faire un corps d'armée constant et reglé. Qu'elle honte!" (III: 12, 1042B/796) [Our armies are no longer bound and held together except by foreign cement; of Frenchmen one can no longer form a steadfast disciplined corps. How shameful!] Personal ambition has replaced discipline and obedience to the leader: "quant à nous, nous nous conduisons à discretion, et non pas du chef, chacun selon la sienne" (1043B/796) [as for ourselves, we follow our own lead and not our leader's, every man in his own way]. For Montaigne, it is the lack of will on the part of the French, a laziness that has allowed the foreign mercenaries to exploit France's internal conflict.

Several decades earlier, Ronsard had lashed out at the bad example set by the Calvinist preachers, who instead of attending Mass and upholding the faith of the country had incited misrule:

> Si tous les predicans eussent vescu ainsi,
> Le peuple ne fust pas, comme il est, en souci,
> Les villes de leurs biens ne seroient despouillées,
> Le laboureur sans crainte eust labouré ses champs,
> . . . .
> Les Reistres, en laissant le rivage du Rhin,
> Comme frelons armez n'eussent beu nostre vin;
> Je me plains de bien peu: ils n'eussent brigandé
> La Gaule qui s'estoit en deux parts desbandée,
> ("Response aux injures," II: 609, vv. 14–18; 22–25)

> If all the preachers had lived this way,
> The people would not, as has happened, so painstakingly
> Plundered all the riches of the cities
> The farmer would have ploughed his fields without fear
> . . . .
> In leaving the banks of the Rhine, the Mercenaries,
> Like hornets would not have drunk our wine;
> I complain of very little: they would not have pillaged
> Gaul divided now into two camps,

D'Aubigné blames external forces, the Medici family, for the violence in France: "Or ne veuille le ciel avoir jugé la France, / A servir septant ans de gibier à Florence, / Ne veuille Dieu tenir pour plus long temps assis, / Sur noz lis tant foulez le joug de Medicis" ("Misères," *Les Tragiques,* I: 305, vv. 797–800) [But let not heaven have condemned France, / To serve seventy years as Florence's prey, / Let God no longer seat / The yoke of the Medici on our trampled lilies]. What for Montaigne had been a failure of will and discipline is for the poet a punishment imposed from without. But both writers agree that France has suffered. Civil conflict, intolerance, and violence, provoked and inflamed by the influence of Rome and Florence has ruined, in the eyes of d'Aubigné, the glory of Paris: "La cité où jadis la loy fut reveree, / Qui à cause des loix fut jadis honoree, / Qui dispensoit en France et la vie et les droicts, / Où fleurissoient les arts" ("Les Fers," *Les Tragiques,* I: 615, 793–96) [The city where formerly the law was revered, / Which because of the law was previously respected, /

Which dispensed in France both life and rights, / In which the arts flourished]. Whether the fault lies with a foreign influence—the Pope or the Medici family—or Frenchmen who massacre their fellow countrymen and women, it is creating discord and conflict between a single people who speak the same language: "Icy les deux partis ne parlent que françois" (615, v. 803). The current conflict is not the French against the Spanish, as in the time of François I; this is a war in which the jailers are the hosts and their own bedrooms are their prisons ("Pour geolier leur hoste, et pour prison leurs chambres"; 616, 814). As Montaigne points out, this is a pestilence that attacks its own body and destroys itself with its own venom: "cette-cy encore contre soy se ronge et se desfaict par son propre venin" (*Les Essais*, III: 12, 1041B/796).

It is perhaps Léry who best expresses the intolerance and violence leading sectors of French society to turn against their own countrymen. As he attacks the act of reducing the town of Sancerre to rubble and of imposing further suffering on the Protestant inhabitants and refugees, he states that the royal forces are winding up the siege by sucking the blood and marrow of its inhabitants: "on achevera de succer le sang et la moëlle" (*Histoire memorable du siège de Sancerre*, 342). The Wars of Religion in France are a vicious act of cannibalism, a kind of sucking of the blood and marrow of the most vulnerable elements of the French population—either those who are under siege or those who are the most vulnerable to attack by soldiers, whether French or foreign. Most importantly, the conflict is on the home turf and leads to acts of fratricide, matricide, and patricide. If Léry lays the blame on the royal troops attacking the innocent inhabitants of Sancerre, Ronsard in his "Response aux injures" accuses the Huguenots for inciting neighbors to kill neighbors, fathers to kill children, and cousins to kill cousins: "le voisin a tué son voisin, / Le pere son enfant, le cousin son cousin?" (*Oeuvres complètes*, II: 602, vv. 24–25). This expanded family conflict has exposed France's frailty to foreign countries and encouraged them to take advantage of the country's weakness. It is indeed the fault of the Calvinists, Ronsard opines, and his Huguenot detractor: "Ou toy, quy en ouvrant le grand cheval de Troye, / As mis tout ce Royaume aux estrangers en proye" (602, vv. 22–23).

Recall that d'Aubigné had described what he calls "maladies implicites" to the sicknesses of "cet Estat," illnesses in which the cure for one organ causes sores in another organ ("Lettre à la Reine Marie de Médicis," *Oeuvres*, II: 196). He states that the Queen Mother has only to enter the patient's room, vial in hand, and administer the medicine. Although the sight and odor are unpleasant, the taste bitter, still the remedy restores to "vie, santé, joye et parfaite guerizon dedans" (196) [life, health, joy and perfect internal healing]. The remedy d'Aubigné suggests is deliberation and consent, along with, as Montaigne had also advised, the return to the first, original, time-honored institution ("rapeler à leur première institution"; 197). D'Aubigné evokes the time of mediation and negotiation, when the courts of Henri III and Henri de Navarre coexisted, and when the freedom of conscience prevailed in many places.

The contrary stance—one that was acted out at Sancerre—was to starve the Huguenots into submission. It is no small wonder that Agrippa d'Aubigné resorts to medical analogies to describe the viciousness of French attacks against her own citizens. As both a witness and a poet chronicling the vicious times, d'Aubigné adopts a metaphor that serves to transmit "a more or less overt message about the attitude the reader [in this case Marie de Medici] should assume" (White, 105). His figurative language orients the Queen Mother and indicates a possible remedy. One is reminded of the physician who treated Henri II and Catherine de Medici, Jean Fernel, and his description of pestilential illnesses, including syphilis:

> Or nous appelons les maladies occultes celles qui proviennent non d'un desordre de tempérament ni de la simple pourriture, mais d'une cause plus cachée qui affecte primitivement et par elle-même toute la substance du corps. . . . Car ce n'est pas, comme le croient la plupart des mornes par la seule pourriture, mais bien par leur nature toute entière et leurs forces destructives, que des causes de cet ordre nous rendent malades ou nous tuent.[4]

> So we call occult diseases those that originate not from a disorder of the temperament or from simple festering but from a hidden cause that infects by itself the very foundation and substance of the body . . . For it is not, as the majority of modern [thinkers] believe, only by the corruption but by their very nature and their destructive forces that the causes of this order makes us sick or kills us.

If in the distant past the French had pulled together against foreign forces—the Spanish or the English, they had in the last century turned against one another in an internal conflict that would kill the body politic as invisible, internal diseases would kill the body. Again, in a letter to Louis XIII, Agrippa d'Aubigné will urge the king not to persecute the

Protestants and to allow them to shed their tears at his feet as they had shed their blood for his father, "Henri le Grand."[5] As Louis's father had prayed in French and fought "en bon François," so too had the Huguenots. D'Aubigné warns Louis XIII that an internal illness threatens him ("un mal au dedans"). It is the cutting tongues ("langues tranchantes") of the hypocrites and flatterers who surround him who risk damning his soul. He bids Louis to honor the agreements that his father had made and maintained and not to hate the religion of his grandmother, Jeanne d'Albret, in which she had brought up Henri IV, Louis's father ("ne briser point les unions que le pere a faites et maintenues," "n'ayez point en execration la Religion où l'excellente Jeanne d'Albret vostre ayeule a nourri, eslevé et instruit son fils"; 614). Like Montaigne, Agrippa d'Aubigné looks back to an era when tolerance reigned and diverging views of spirituality coexisted among those at the highest levels of influence. It was in such a period that the arts flourished along with the citizens, when each individual contributed to the glory of France.

The effect of the French Wars of Religion on the social fabric of France was clear to those who were involved both in the artistic as well as the diplomatic affairs of the early modern period. Present from the very outset of both the outbreak of syphilis and the first signs of persecution against those who espoused Reform ideology, Erasmus could indeed have applied the words he penned about syphilis to the steady debilitating force of religious intolerance in France: "*This* disease is simply slow but sure death, or rather burial" (CWE, 40: 853). It would be centuries before the country would recover from the loss of life and productive intellectual and physical force that came about during the years of civil and religious conflict in France. And yet, as in Théodore de Bèze's *Abraham sacrifiant,* the Huguenots are left to witness the suffering of their martyrs—their faith as a model of "la vive foy." Dating from 1550, as the conflict is only heating up and the terrible massacres of innocents—Catholic and Protestant—lie ahead, the epilogue warns the reader to stand to witness the faith and courage of an Abraham given his son Isaac and then asked to sacrifice him:

> Or toy grand Dieu, qui nous as faict cognoistre
> Les grans abuz esquels nous voyons estre
> Le povre monde, helas, tant perverty,
> Fay qu'un chacun de nous soit adverty
> En son endroit, de tourner en usage
> La vive foy de ce sainct personnage.[6]

> So you, great God, who reveals to us
> The huge abuses which we see to be
> The wretched world, alas, so corrupted,
> Warn every one of us
> Where we are, to put to good use
> The living faith of this holy being [Abraham].

The witnessing at once alerts the Huguenots to the fact that they have, like Abraham, been constant to their "vive foy," but it also reminds them that like Abraham, they are confused by the enormity of the sacrifice asked: turning against their countrymen, exile, severe hunger that tests their human values against cannibalism. For the Huguenots who witness the countless massacres and persecution of their people, it is clear that their faith has been tested well beyond the limits of human reason: "Par la bonté de Dieu, ha la foy telle, / Que nonobstant toute raison humaine, / Jamais de Dieu la parolle n'est vaine" (*Abraham sacrifiant,* 87, vv. 924–26) [By God's goodness, faith is such / That not withstanding all human reason, / God's word is never without purpose]. For the Catholics, witnessing takes another form. Observing the starvation, loss of life, and pervasive breakdown in the rule of law, the voices of reason saw, toward the end of the century, that giving in to the most extreme voices on either side of the conflict had weakened France to the point that recovery depended on finding a compromise and return to peace. The metaphor of disease and the rhetoric of the pox dissipated as opposing parties realized that for the survival of France itself, it was vital to restore order, communication, and understanding. Topical remedies had to be supplanted by systemic cures.

NOTES

PREFACE AND ACKNOWLEDGMENTS

1. Michel de Montaigne, *Les Essais,* ed. Pierre Villey (Paris: Presses Universitaires de France, 1992), II, 37, 772A. All citations in French for Montaigne will refer to this edition and in English to the translation of Donald Frame, *The Complete Essays of Montaigne,* trans. Donald M. Frame (Stanford: Stanford University Press, 1965), II, 37, 585–86.

INTRODUCTION

1. André Thevet, *Histoire d'André Thevet Angoumousin, cosmographe du Roy, de deux voyages faits aux Indes Australes et Occidentales,* ed. Jean-Claude Laborie et Frank Lestringant (Geneva: Droz, 2006), 211. Among chroniclers, humanists writing in Latin and in the vernacular, and physicians, it became apparent very early that syphilis was sexually transmitted, as shall be seen here and in later chapters. What is curious is that Fracastor, whose shepherd Syphilus or Syphile would give his name to the disease in later centuries, attributes the transmission to the air and not to sexual relations with men or women already infected with the disease. Fracastor describes how the vast spaces of air are filled with the pollution and an unknown filth spreads its contagion throughout the air: "Paulatim aerij tractus et inania lata / accepere luem uacuasque insuetus in auras / marco iji coelumque tulit contagi in omne," Jérôme Fracastor, *La Syphilis ou le mal français / Syphilis sive morbus gallicus,* trans. Jacqueline Vons (Paris: Les Belles Lettres, 2011), I: vv. 247–49. Vons notes that it is indeed remarkable that Fracastor omits mention of the sexual transmission of the pox from the first book of his celebrated work, Fracastor LXIII. Jean Fernel, court physician to Henri II and Diane de Poitiers, among others, could not be more blunt in attributing the transmission of the pox to sexual intercourse: "Il [le mal vénérien/Lues Venerea] se contracte seulement par le coït ou par quelque autre contact impur," Jean Fernel d'Amiens, *Le Meilleur traitement du Mal Vénérien* 1579, trans. L. Le Pileur (Paris: G. Masson, 1879), ch. 1, 3.

2. Jean de Léry, *Histoire d'un voyage faict en la terre du Brésil*, 2nd ed., ed. Frank Lestringrant (Paris: Le Livre de Poche, 1994), 469: "Ils ont une maladie terrible qu'ils nomment Pians."

3. Francesco Guerra, "The Problem of Syphilis," in *First Images of America: The Impact of the New World on the Old*, ed. Fredi Chiappelli et al. (Berkeley: University of California Press, 1976), 2: 845–51. A recent article, called to my attention by Plymouth State University anthropologist Katherine C. Donahue, reveals that modern genomic sequencing in 1998 confirms the "convention of dividing the bacterium into three subspecies: *T. pallidum* subspecies *pallidum* (syphilis), *T. pallidum* subspecies pertenue (yaws), and *T. pallidum* subspecies endemicum (bejel)." Yet the subspecies are remarkably similar. The researchers have not found a single case with a corresponding reliable date and clear evidence of treponemal skeletal lesions that demonstrates the presence of syphilis in Europe prior to Columbus's return from the New World. See Kristin N. Harper, Molly K. Zuckerman, and George J. Armelagos, "Syphilis: Then and Now," *The Scientist Magazine*, February 1, 2014, 1–8, http.//www.the-scientist.com/TheScientist/daily/2014/02/05a.html.

4. Anthony Pagden, *The Fall of Natural Man: The American Indian and the Origins of Comparative Ethnology* (Cambridge: Cambridge University Press, 1986), 86. Cited by William Eamon, "Cannibalism and Contagion: Framing Syphilis in Counter-Reformation Italy," *Early Science and Medicine* 3, no. 1 (1998): 18.

5. William Eamon, 10. Eamon references Fioravanti's work, *Capricci medicinali* (Venice, 1582), originally published in 1561: "Thus the armies of both sides, having so many times eaten human flesh, began to be polluted in such a way that not a single man remained who was not full of sores and pains, and the majority became bald" (49v).

6. Vons quotes Dr. L. Pileur in stating that *gorre* is not related to sow (*la gorre/la truie*) but to *goir*, meaning pustules, open pus-filled sores, XXX–XXXI. See "Gorre et grande gorre," *Bulletin de la Société de l'Histoire de la Médicine* 9 (1910): 217–24, cited by Vons in her introduction to Fracastor's work.

7. See the variant spelling, *grosse vairolle*, in the title of Thierry de Héry's *La Méthode curatoire pour la maladie vénérienne, vulgairement appelée grosse vairolle, et de la diversité des ses symptomes* (Paris: Matthieu David et Arnoud L'Angelier, 1552), cited by Vons XXVIII.

8. Henry Heller, "Marguerite de Navarre, and the Reformers of Meaux," *Bibiliothèque d'Humanisme et Renaissance* 33, no. 2 (1971): 271–310; Ehsan Ahmed, "Guillaume Briçonnet, Marguerite de Navarre and the Evangelical Critique of Reason," *Bibliothèque d'Humanisme et Renaissance* 69, no. 3 (2007): 615–25.

9. Guillaume Briçonnet and Marguerite d'Angoulême, *Correspondance (1521–1524)*, 2 vols., ed. Christine Martineau and Michel Veissière (Geneva: Droz, 1975 and 1979), I: 172 (letter of February 26, 1522).

10. Denis Crouzet, *La nuit de la Saint-Bathélemy: Un rêve perdu de la Renaissance* (Paris: Pluriel, 2012), 17.

11. R. J. Knecht, *The French Wars of Religion 1559–1598*, 2nd ed. (London: Longman, 1996), 3.

12. Barbara B. Diefendorf, *The Saint Bartholomew's Day Massacre. A Brief History with Documents* (Boston: Bedford/St. Martin's, 2009), 13–14: "Once again, however, Catherine's attempt at compromise offended people on both sides of the religious divide. Protestants complained that their right to worship was still too limited, while Catholics were outraged that any worship was permitted at all" (13).

13. François López de Gómara, *Histoire générale des Indes occidentales et terres neuves, qui iusques à present esté descouvertes, augmentée en cest cinquiesme édition*

de la description de la nouvelle Espagne de de la grande ville de Mexiques, autrement nommé, Tenuctilan, composée en espagnol par François López de Gómara, et traduicte en François par S. de Genillé Mart. Fumée. À Paris chez Michel Sonnius, rue sainct Jacques, à l'enseigne de l'escu de Basle, M. D. LXXXVII; 40r°. López de Gómara states: "Au commencement ce mal estoit bien violent, infect, & deshonneste: mais aujourd'hui il n'est si rigoureux, ne si deshonneste" [In the beginning this illness was very violent, infectious, and filthy: but today it is not so severe, nor as foul].

14. Michel de Montaigne, *Les Essais,* ed. Pierre Villey, 3 vols. (Paris: Presses Universitaires de France, 1992), II: ch. 37, 772. All citations in French will refer to this edition, and in English to the translation of Donald Frame: *The Complete Essays of Montaigne,* trans. Donald M. Frame (Stanford: Stanford University Press, 1965), 586.

15. Agrippa d'Aubigné, *Les Tragiques,* ed. Jean-Raymond Fanlo, 2 vols. (Paris: Honoré Champion, 2003), I: 267, v. 97.

16. Michel Foucault, *Les mots et les choses* (Paris: Gallimard, 1966), 32.

17. In *Sampling the Book: Renaissance Prologues and the French Conteurs* (Lewisburg, PA: Bucknell University Press, 1994), I examine Foucault's discussion of likeness in the context of prefatory metaphors (46–47).

18. Joel Fineman, "The History of the Anecdote: Fiction and Fiction," in *The New Historicism,* ed. H. Aram Veeser (New York: Routledge, 1989), 55.

19. Agrippa d'Aubigné, *Oeuvres,* ed. Jean-Raymond Fanlo, 2 vols. (Paris: Honoré Champion, 2007), II: 196.

20. Hayden White, *Tropics of Discourse: Essays in Cultural Criticism* (Baltimore: Johns Hopkins University Press, 1985), 46.

21. John Henderson, *The Renaissance Hospital: Healing the Body and Healing the Soul* (New Haven, CT: Yale University Press, 2006), 113–15.

22. Rudolph Arbesmann, "The Concept of 'Christus Medicus' in St. Augustine," *Traditio* 10 (1954): 9–10.

23. *Recueil de poésies françoises des XVe et XVIe siècles. Morales, facétieuses, historiques,* ed. Anatole de Montaiglon, I (Paris: P. Jannet, 1855), 72.

24. François Rabelais, *Le Quart Livre faits et dits héroïques du bon Pantagruel,* in *Oeuvres complètes,* ed. Guy Demerson (Paris: Éditions du Seuil, 1973), 580: "S'il plaist au bon Dieu, vous obtiendrez santé."

25. Léry, *Histoire d'un voyage,* 176–77; for the English translation of Léry's work I cite Jean de Léry, *History of a Voyage to the Land of Brazil,* trans. Janet Whatley (Berkeley: University of California Press, 1992), 41.

26. *Satyres chrestiennes de la cuisine papale,* ed. Charles-Antoine Chamay (Geneva: Droz, 2005), Satyre V, 105, v. 384.

27. Artus Désiré, *Le contrepoison des cinquante-dix chansons de Clément Marot,* ed. Jacques Pineaux (Geneva: Droz, 1977), Chanson XXXXIIII, 50; Chanson XXVI, 40.

28. *Oeuvres complètes,* ed. Gustave Cohen, 2 vols. (Paris: Gallimard, 1950): 551–73.

29. Erasmus, *Colloquies, Collected Works of Erasmus,* trans. Craig R. Thompson (Toronto: The University of Toronto Press, 1997), 40: 689: "Certainly France, nay the whole world, might thus be bound in friendship. For if the sore is covered up by bad terms rather than truly healed, I fear that when the wound is opened on some occasion soon afterwards, the old poison may burst out with more harm than ever."

30. Marjorie O'Rourke Boyle, "Erasmus' Prescription for Henry VIII: Logotherapy," *Renaissance Quarterly* 31, no. 2 (1978): 161–72. She quotes Erasmus's letter of advice to Henry VIII, *Erasmi epistolae,* ed. P. S. Allen et al. (Oxford: Oxford University Press, 1906–53), V, 318, ll. 250–51.

31. D'Aubigné, *Oeuvres,* II: 230.

32. D'Aubigné, *Oeuvres*: "Voylà pourquoy j'appeloys les malladies de cet Estat implicites quand le remede de l'un ulcere l'autre" (II: 196).

33. I note the recent discovery of a manuscript by Ingrid De Smet of a manuscript from Montaigne's library, signed "Michaël Montanus," and containing notes from a course on Roman law given by the legal scholar and historian François Baudouin. See "Un manuscrit de François Baudouin dans la librairie de Montaigne," *Bibliothèque d'Humanisme et Renaissance* 75 (2013): 105–11. Baudouin's position as a "moyenneur," in favor of peace between the Catholics and Protestants at the failed *colloque de Poissy* in February 1561, mirrors Montaigne's view that the tolerant state where justice rules is a healthy state. Discipline, whether in the individual's or the army's willingness to heed the law, creates a prosperous and healthy country. When jurisprudence fails, when each person takes the law into his or her own hands, the kingdom reeks of infection. In speaking of the monstrous religious and civil conflict in which France had been engaged for much of his lifetime, Montaigne depicts the conflict eating away at its own body: "Monstrueuse guerre: les autres agissent au dehors; cette-cy encore contre soys e ronge et se desfaict par son propre venin.... Toute discipline la fuyt. Elle vient guarir la sedition et en est pleine" (*Les Essais*, III: 12, 1041B/796) [Monstrous war! Other wars act outward; this one acts also against itself, eats and destroys itself by its own venom.... All discipline flies from it. It comes to cure sedition and is full of it]. For both Baudouin and Montaigne, the health of the kingdom depended on respect for the law.

CHAPTER 1

1. "Un *corps en mouvement*," "n'est jamais *prêt* ni *achevé*," "*est toujours en état de construction, de création et lui-même construit un autre corp*" (emphasis is Bakhtin's). Mikhail Bakhtin, *Rabelais and His World*, trans. Hélène Iswolsky (Cambridge, MA: MIT Press, 1968), 317; Mikhaïl Bakhtine, *L'oeuvre de François Rabelais et la culture populaire au moyen âge et sous la renaissance*, trans. Andrée Robel (Paris: Gallimard, 1970), 315.

2. E. Jeanselme, *Histoire de la syphilis. Son origine. Son expansion. Progrès realisés dans l'étude de cette maladie depuis la fin du XVe siècle jusqu'à l'époque contemporaine. Extrait du Traité de la syphilis*, vol. 1 (Paris: G. Doin, 1931), 121. Jeanselme notes that Gasparis Torella (also spelled Gaspare Torrella) observed the secondary infection passed to babies from wet nurses or nursing mothers as early as 1500 in his *Dialogus de dolore, cum tractactu de ulceribus in pudendagra evenire solitis* (Impressus per Joannem Besicken & Martinum de Amsterdam, 1500). Jeanselme comments that Torella witnessed nurses with pustules on their breasts or face breastfeeding or kissing young babies. Torella states that the child's infection is a secondary infection passed on from the nurse, whose disease was a primary infection. For a very complete discussion of the consequences of having healthy wet nurses from the Italian mountainous, rural areas nurse babies born most often of prostitutes infected with syphilis, see David Kertzner, *Amalia's Tale (*Boston: Houghton Mifflin, 2008). Set in the nineteenth century, the story of Amalia Bagnacavalli's struggle, through her lawyer Augusto Barbieri, to seek redress and compensation in the courts documents the dangers of contracting syphilis through nursing infant children.

3. Jeanselme, *Histoire*, 106: "La vérole n'épargne aucune condition sociale. Tous les hommes, depuis tous le plus élevé juqu'au plus humble, sont égaux devant elle." He goes on to cite prominent victims: Pope Alexander VI, Cardinal Jean Borgia, King Francois I, the knight Ulrich von Hutten, and the goldsmith Benvenuto Cellini.

4. See L. W. Harrison, "The Origin of Syphilis," *British Journal of Venereal Diseases* 35, no. 1 (1959): 1–7.

5. Fernel d'Amiens, *Le Meilleur traitement du Mal Vénérien*. This is a French translation of *De Luës Venerea curatione perfectissima Liber*, an edition published posthumously in 1579.

6. Rabelais, *Oeuvres complètes*, 213. François Rabelais, *The Complete Works of François Rabelais*, trans. Donald M. Frame (Berkeley: University of California Press, 1991), 133. All quotations and French and English translations will refer to these two editions.

7. *Satyres chrestiennes de la cuisine papale*, 47, vv. 159–60.

8. Fracastor (Hieronymus Fracastorius), *La Syphilis ou le mal français*, Liber II, 47, vv. 236–40: "Interea si membra dolor conuulsa malignus / torqueat, oesypo propera lenire dolorem / mastichinoque oleo, lentum quibus anseris unguen, / emulsumque potes lini de semine mucum, / narcissumque, inulamque, liquentiaque addere mella." Vons's French translation is extremely readable and provides an excellent and extensive introduction. The *editio princeps* was published in 1530, following unauthorized versions made when a version of the first two books sent to Pietro Bembo for comments fell into the wrong hands (*La Syphilis*, XLVI–LI). Fracastoro went on to add the third book, in which he develops the fable around the naming of the disease and, just as importantly, the praise of guaiac wood as the saving remedy for both indigenous people of the New World and Europeans later.

9. Ulrich von Hutten, *De l'expérience et approbation Ulrich de Hutten notable chevalier touchant la medecine du boys dict guiacum pour circonvenir et deschasser lamaladie indeuement appellee françoise. Aincoys par gens de meilleur urgent est dicte et appelee la maladie de Naples traduicte et interpretee par maistre Jehan Cheradame hypocrates estudiant en la faculté et art de medecine*, in-4° (Paris: Jean Trepperel, n.d.), ch. 7. In his article "The Aggression of the Cured Syphilitic: Ulrich von Hutten's Projections of His Disease as Metaphor," *The German Quarterly* 68, no. 1 (Winter 1995): 1–18, Lewis Jillings states that Hutten underwent his treatment in September to October 1518.

10. Ambroise Paré, *Oeuvres complètes*, ed. J.-F. Malgaigne, 3 vols. (Geneva: Slatkine Reprints, 1970), II: 540.

11. *Opera omnia*, ed. Eduard Böcking (Leipzig, 1859–1870), IV: 27–41. Jillings notes that it was "written probably in Augsburg, published in Mainz by Johann Schöffer in February 1519," and translated perhaps by Martin Bucer in 1519 (16, n. 42). While effective treatments for syphilis are not really the subject of this book, it is well known that Hutten made famous the use of guaiacum or holy wood, a treatment later commented on by the chroniclers back from the New World, such as Jean de Léry. See my article "The Old World Meets the New in Montaigne's *Essais*: The Nexus of Syphilis, Cannibalism, and Empirical Medicine," *Montaigne Studies* 22, nos. 1–2 (2010): 85–100.

12. In his recent article "From *Satura* to *Satyre*: François Rabelais and the Renaissance Appropriation of a Genre," *Renaissance Quarterly* 67, no. 2 (Summer 2014): 377–424, Bernd Renner shows the evolution of satire from the more ludic, less scathing Horatian satire typical of the first half of the sixteenth century and of Rabelais's *Pantagruel* and *Gargantua* to the more biting, "punishing" satire characteristic of Juvenal which took hold in France as the religious wars progressed (390–91).

13. As will be evident in chapters 5 and 6 of this book, discipline is a theme taken up by several literary giants of the second half of the century, such as Montaigne and Agrippa d'Aubigné, who also advanced the countersuggestion that the absence of discipline weakened the health of the kingdom.

14. Grace Q. Vicary, "Visual Art as Social Data: The Renaissance Codpiece," *Cultural Anthropology* 4, no. 1 (February 1989), 8.

15. Elizabeth Rodini, "Functional Jewels," *Art Institute of Chicago Museum Studies* 25, no. 2 (2000): 76–78, 108.

16. See François Rigolot's article on this episode, in which he compares Panurge's three attempts to seduce the "haulte dame de Paris" wtih St. Matthew's recounting of Satan's temptation of Christ, "Rabelais, Misogyny, and Christian Charity: Biblical Intertextuality and the Renaissance Crisis of Exemplarity," *PMLA* 109, no. 2 (March 1994): 225–37.

17. Citing Judson B. Gilbert's *Disease and Destiny: A Bibliography of Medical Reference* (London: Dawsons, 1962), Vicary states that "it is possible each of them [François I, Charles V, and Henry VIII] had acquired syphilis in their youth and their tailors, or physicians, had suggested they adopt the artifact worn by soldiers" (18). See also Katherine Crawford, *The Sexual Culture of the French Renaissance* (Cambridge: Cambridge University Press, 2010), 202. She speculates that François I "probably" contracted syphilis by 1524 and suffered from it until his death. In her recent book *Blood Will Tell: A Medical Explanation of the Tyranny of Henry VIII* (Bloomington, IA: Ashwood Press, 2012), Kyra Cornelius Kramer advances the theory that Henry VIII did not suffer from syphilis but rather from the inheritance of the Kell positive blood type, known to cause fetal and newborn mortality as well as McLeod syndrome, provoking both debilitating psychological and physical problems such as those from which the king was known to suffer (chapter 1).

18. Rudolph Arbesmann notes eight examples from St. Augustine's sermon that reference Christus medicus, "the notion of Christ as healer of man's spiritual diseases," "The Concept of Christus Medicus in St. Augustine," 1–28. In his article "The Sorbonnic Trots: Staging the Intestinal Distress of the Roman Catholic Church in French Reform Theater," *Renaissance Quarterly* 56, no. 4 (Winter 2003): 1089–111, Jeff Persels brings up the image of Christus medicus in the context of illness as metaphor in French reform theater.

19. These attributes of the physician are present in the "ancien prologue" to the abbreviated version of the fourth book published in 1548 (771).

20. Boyle, "Erasmus' Prescription for Henry VIII," 165. She paraphrases parts of Erasmus's letter to Henry of 1523, *Erasmi epistolae*, ed. P. S. Allen et al., 12 vols (Oxford: Oxford University Press, 1906–53), V: 316, ll. 129–34.

21. Margaret Healy, "Bronzino's London Allegory and the Art of Syphilis," *Oxford Art Journal* 20, no. 1 (1997): 6.

22. Erasmus, *Erasmi Epistolae*, 1789c. Cited by Healy, 6.

23. See Deborah N. Losse, "Revisioning Saint Augustine: Rabelaisian Intertexts of Augustine's *Confessions*," *Allegorica* 23 (2002): 19–31: "Panurge is clearly troubled by a divided will, where he cannot be receptive to the signs that God gives him because he is a slave to passion. His will is divided. Augustine describes his own state of mind before conversion" (26). Augustine expresses the dilemma in these terms: "Ita duae uoluntates meae, una uetus, alia noua, illa carnalis, illa spiritalis, confligebant inter se atque discordando dissipabant animam meam" (*Confessions*, VIII, v, 10) [So these two wills within me, one old, one new, one the servant of the flesh, the other of the spirit, were in conflict and between them they tear my soul apart]. The Latin citation is taken from Saint Augustine, *Confessions*, ed. Pierre de Labriolle, 2 vols. (Paris: Les Belles Lettres, 1994); the English translation from Saint Augustine, trans. R. S. Pine-Coffin, *Confessions* (London: Penguin Books, 1961).

24. Gargantua's remonstration against the Church's involvement in clandestine marriages undertaken without the parents' knowledge (ch. 48, *Le Tiers Livre*) is one illustration of the importance of the parental role. A second illustration is found in the colloquy "A Marriage In Name Only Or An Unequal Marriage" (Erasmus, *Colloquies*, 40: 843–59), discussed in chapter 2 of this book, in which Erasmus rebukes the parents who married their daughter to an inappropriately old and syphilitic man. They have simply ignored their parental duty to select a suitable spouse for their daughter.

CHAPTER 2

1. Franz Bierlaire, *Les Colloques d'Érasme: réforme des études, réforme des moeurs et réforme de l'Eglise au XVIe siècle* (Paris: Les Belles Lettres, 1978), 80: "Tout ce qui survient dans sa vie quotidienne s'y mêle." Huizinga states that Erasmus was probably born in 1466, although "the illegitimacy of his birth has thrown a veil of mystery over his descent and kinship," J. Huizinga, *Erasmus of Rotterdam* (New York: Phaidon Publishers, 1952), 5.

2. Barbara Cornell, "Malleable Material, Models of Power: Women in Erasmus's 'Marriage Group' and Civility in Boys," *ELH* 57, no. 2 (Summer 1990): 243.

3. When the English translation of the Latin text of the *Colloquies* is cited, the work referenced will be *Collected Works of Erasmus* (abbreviated CWE). For the Latin text of the *Familiarium colloquiorum formulae* or *Colloquia*, the *Opera Omnia Desiderii Erasmi Roterodami*, I–3 (abbreviated OO) will be used (Amsterdam: The New Holland Press, 1969).

4. See Eva Kushner, "Les Colloques et l'inscription de l'autre dans le discours," in *Dix conférences sur Érasme. Éloge de la folie—Colloques*, ed. Claude Blum (Paris/Geneva: Honoré Champion, 1988), 33–47. In his insightful article "The Mimesis of Marriage: Dialogue and Intimacy in Erasmus's Matrimonial Writings," *Renaissance Quarterly* 57, no. 4 (Winter 2004): 1278–1307, Reinier Leushuis cites Kushner's view of the diverse origins of the Erasmian dialogue: "Erasmus adopts in the *Colloquies* a mixture of the characteristics of the harmonious Ciceronian model (where, after a brief introduction or *narratio*, two or more characters discuss . . . the argument they stand for in order to emphasize the more persuasive one), the dissymmetrical Socratic model (with the predominance of a Socratic voice that seeks to lead the interlocutor step-by-step to the truth), and the Lucianic model (characterized by its vivacious and satirical exchange)," (1295). In *Less Rightly Said: Scandals and Readers in Sixteenth-Century France* (Stanford: Stanford University Press, 2010), Antonia Szabari refers to Erasmus's "lowering of the tone" as a "corrective device" (11). Turning to Lucianic satire "as a mask to mitigate the offensive potential of an utterance," Erasmus seeks to correct in lighter, amusing manner, one that is more effective than assuming a stern, overbearing voice. While his *modus loquendi* did not always assuage the anger of the censors nor of readers opposed to his point of view, Szabari points out that this satirical mask "proves to be effective in converting French humanists to anti-Catholic reformed ideas" (12).

5. Kushner, "Un récit d'une conversation orientée vers une solution," 21; Rudolf Hirzel, *Der Dialog, Ein Literarhistorischen Versuch* (Leipzig: S. Hirzel, 1895).

6. It should be noted that Erasmus added five dialogues (not related to the theme) to another edition published in 1531, as well as two more dialogues to the edition published in 1533—this last the final edition overseen by its author and widely reprinted (OO, introduction, 14–15).

7. Jeanselme, *Histoire de la syphilis*, 63–65. Citing from Oviedo's *Historia general y natural* (volume 1, book II, chapter 7, p. 28), Jeanselme quotes Oviedo stating that when the armies of Charles VIII met the Spanish armies, the sickness passed from the Spanish to the French and Italian soldiers (65). Oviedo observes that this was the first time that the sickness had been seen in Italy ("c'est la première fois qu'on la vit en Italie"). Oviedo notes as well that since it was at the time that the French soldiers arrived with Charles, the Italians called the sickness the French disease ("et comme c'était à l'époque où les Français vinrent avec le dit roi Charles, les Italiens appèlerent cette maladie le mal Françès"; 65).

8. In his formal study of the *Colloquiorum Familiarium formulae*, Franz Bierlaire attributes a more one-sided contest between the Carthusian and soldier than does Kushner, but Bierlaire is correct in stating that the Carthusian sweeps away the soldier's arguments one by one: "Le chartreux balaie un à un tous les arguments antimonastiques du soldat," *Érasme et ses colloques: Le livre d'une vie* (Geneva: Droz, 1977), 66.

9. "Depuis la reprise des hostilités entre Charles-Quint et François Ier, il n'a pas cessé de pousser des cris d'alarme" (*Érasme et ses colloques*, 66).

10. Franz Bierlaire notes the parallel, drawn by Erasmus, between the youth's reading of Erasmus's edition of the New Testament and the young man's efforts to successfully persuade the prostitute to reform her life, much as in the conversion of Thaïs by the hermit Paphnuce. It is part of the Erasmian goal to inspire youth to embrace modesty and to turn away from whoring (*Érasme et ses colloques*, 68–69).

11. Much as Marguerite de Navarre would later amuse the readers by inscribing her persona in the *Heptaméron*, Erasmus inscribed his own edition of the New Testament (1516) in Greek, and his Latin translation is based on the Greek text, which the young man takes along with him on his trip to Rome. Lucretia notes that some label Erasmus "more than a heretic." To which the young man states: "You don't mean that man's reputation has reached this place?" CWE, 39: 384). This bantering allows Lucretia to note that his name and reputation as a heretic have come to her through her clients of the gown—the priests who frequent the brothel. These clergy, no doubt ignorant of Greek and so unable to question his new Latin translation, follow the Church's view that Erasmus is in league with Luther, presumably because his reliance on the Greek manuscripts of the New Testament leads him to omit mention of the Trinity in the opening of 1 John 5:7: "There are three that bear record in heaven: the Father, the Word, and the Holy Spirit, and these are three in one." See George Huntston Williams, *The Radical Reformation*, 3rd ed. (Kirksville, MO: Truman State University Press, 2000), 43. Erasmus's satirical view of corrupt and poorly educated clergy comes through in his self-inscription in the colloquy.

12. In a letter to Erasmus, François Rabelais alludes to this same care that the expectant mother takes to shelter her unborn child, here referred to as a seed within her that she has never seen. He likens the natural maternal love to the care and nurturing that Erasmus has provided Rabelais, even though Erasmus has never seen the physician's face nor known his name; see *La Correspondance d'Érasme*, trans. P. S. Allen, H. M. Allen, and H. W. Garrod (Bruxelles: University Press, 1981), 10: 170.

13. Valerie Fildes, *Wet Nursing: A History from Antiquity to the Present* (Oxford: Blackwell Press, 1988), 69. Critical for my purposes as an influence on Erasmian views are the German surgeons Bartholomaeus Metlinger and Eucharias Roesslin and the Swiss Felix Wurtz—all writing at the end of the fifteenth or beginning of the sixteenth centuries.

14. In his book *Lost Girls: Sex and Death in Renaissance Florence* (Baltimore: Johns Hopkins University Press, 2010), Nicholas Terpstra explores the deaths of very young women who were brought to the Casa della Pietà in Florence at an early age, either because they were orphaned or, more usually, abandoned by their parents (151). He suspects syphilis to have been a principal cause.

15. Montaigne, *Les Essais*, II: 8, 399. In this essay, "De l'affection des pères aux enfans," addressed to madame d'Éstissac, who was the widow of Jean d'Estissac, Montaigne resumes a theme in the colloquy between Fabulla and Eutrapelus—that mothers are best suited to nourish children in the first years before the father assumes the education of the child's mind. Eutrapelus lets Fabulla know that when she states she is less concerned with the formation of the body of her child than with his mind, she speaks "piously" but not "philosophically," because it is the father's role to form the child's mind: "There will come a time, a grace of God, when you will send away your young son from you out of doors to be accomplished with learning and undergo harsh discipline, and which indeed is rather the province of the father than of the mother, but now its tender age calls for indulgence" (229). Montaigne also decries the injustice of the practice of sending children to the wet nurse, in that the children of the wet nurse suffer from being separated from their mothers so that the mothers can serve as wet nurses to the noblewomen. Like Erasmus, he acknowledges the "natural" bond between the mother and the child but laments the fact that in his century, such natural bonds have weakened: "Au demeurant, il est aisé à voir par experience que cette affection naturelle, à qui nous donnons tant d'authorité, a les racines bien foibles" (II: 8, 399).

16. Rabelais, *Oeuvres complètes*, *Gargantua*, ch. 7, 58.

17. Rabelais, *The Complete Works*, 21. "Car de trouver nourrice suffisante n'estoit possible en tout le pays, considéré la grande quantité de laict requis pour icelluy alimenter, combien qu'aulcuns docteurs scotistes ayent affermé que sa mère alaicta et qu'elle pouvoit traire de ses mammelles quatorze cens deux pipes neuf potées de laict pour chascune foys, ce que n'est vraysemblable, et esté la proposition déclairée mammallement scandaleuse, des pityoyable aureilles offensive, et sentent de loing hérésie" (ch. 7, 58).

18. Bierlaire reports that on May 16, 1526, theologians had declared that children were not to read the *Colloquies* because the dialogues were a corrupting force (*Les Colloques d'Érasme*, 217).

19. Bierlaire speculates on the identity for Pompilius Blenus, stating that he is certainly a composite of aging syphilitics. Chief among the names proposed for creating the composite portrait of the aging syphilitic who marries a youthful beauty are Henri von Eppendorf, Ulrich von Hutten, and Thomas Brun (*Érasme et ses colloques*, 100). Iphigenia as a tragic figure would have been recognized by all readers of the *Colloquies*.

20. An anonymous poem, "La complainte de Messire Pierre Liset sur le trespas de son feu nez" refers to the pock-ridden former president of the Parlement de Paris, who had banned many Protestants from Paris for heresy. See [Théodore de Bèze], *Satyres chrestiennes de la cuisine papale*, 162–67.

21. Rabelais, *Oeuvres complètes*, *Le Tiers Livre*, ch. 48, 442/401; Marguerite de Navarre, *L'Heptaméron*, ed. Michel François (Paris: Garnier Frères, 1967), 158–75.

22. Cited by Leushuis, "The Mimesis of Marriage," 1290. CWE, 25: 139; OO, I-5, 399–400: "Quod enim dulcius quam cum ea vivere cum qua sis non benevolentiae modo, verumetiam corporum mutua quadam communione arctissime copulatus?"

23. I am reminded of Grandgousier's failure to understand the bellicose intentions of Picrochole and his desire for world conquest in Rabelais's *Gargantua*. Writing to his son

Gargantua to urge him to return home, Grandgousier shows what measures he has taken to persuade Picrochole to make peace: "My intention is not to provoke, but to appease; not to attack, but to defend, not to conquer, but to protect my loyal subjects and hereditary lands, which Picrochole has invaded without cause or occasion, and from day to day pursues his mad enterprise with excesses intolerable to free men" (*Complete Works*, 71). "Ma déliberation n'est de provocquer, ains de dapaiser; d'assaillir, mais défendre; de conquester, mais de guarder mes féaulx subjectz et terres héréditaires és quelles est hostillement entré Picrochole sans cause et occasion, et de jour en jour poursuit sa furieuse entrprinse avecques excès non tolérable à personnes libères" (*Oeuvres complètes*, 133). The two interlocutors evoke the captivity of François I after the battle of Pavia (February 24, 1525), and this mention permits us to date the passage from between February 1525 and 1526. Erasmus corresponded with both Charles V and François I. He wrote to François I on his return to Paris in a letter dated June 16, 1526, and spoke of the public joy on the end of hostilities between the two rivals. See CWE, 40: 731, n. 89.

24. Medical metaphors were not unknown to Erasmus. In explaining his vast revisions of the much smaller 1518 and 1519 unauthorized versions of the *Formulae*, the humanist comments on his revisions: "Voyant cette oeuvre accueillie des écoliers avec le vif enthousiasme . . . je fis servir cet engouement au progrès des études. *Les médecins n'accordent pas toujours aux malades les aliments les plus salubres; ils leur permettent quelquefois ceux qui excitent davantage leur appétit*" (emphasis added); *De utilitate colloquiorum*, in OO, I: 3, 123, cited by Bierlaire, *Érasme et ses colloques*, 33.

25. Writing *Syphilis sive morbus gallicus* (1530) at roughly the same time, Girolamo Fracastoro (Hieronymus Fracastorius) creates an epic version in which is suggested the link between the violence waged in territorial expansion with the outbreak of syphilis. In his heroic poem, the Spanish soldiers' shooting down the birds in the New World and invading the lands of peaceful indigenous peoples there bring on the vengeance of the gods and eventually lead to the spread of the dreaded unknown disease to Europe. Fracastoro describes a bird, speaking for Apollo, foreseeing the future wars and deaths of the Spanish: "Sed non ante nouas dabitur summittere terras, / et longa populos in libertate quietos, / molirique urbes, ritusque ac sacra nouare, / quam uos infandos pelagi terraeque labores / perpessi, diuersa hominum post praelia, multi / mortua in externa tumuletis corpora terra" [But you will not have a chance to subjugate the new lands nor their inhabitants who have lived there so long, nor to establish cities or your religious rites and sacred ceremonies before many among you have endured horrible suffering on land and sea, fought with foreigners, and buried dead bodies in foreign land], Fracastor, *La Syhilis ou le mal français*, Liber III, 71, vv. 179–84 (my translation from the Latin).

26. See Boyle, "Erasmus' Prescription for Henry VIII," 161–72. She quotes Erasmus's letter of advice to Henry VIII, *Erasmi epistolae*, ed. P. S. Allen et al., 12 vols. (Oxford: Oxford University Press, 1906–53), V: 318-19, ll. 251–71. She shows how Erasmus encourages Henry VIII to put his faith in the word of God through Christ and so to pursue peace rather than war (169).

27. See Bierlaire, *Les Colloques d' Érasme*: "C'est dans la rue qu'Érasme choisit ses personnages et c'est le plus souvent dans la rue qu'il les fait se rencontrer" (79). Evangelical humanists, such as Bonaventure des Périers, continue to highlight the wisdom of the common people, as in the case of the herring seller ("la belle harangere") who takes on the learned regent on the Petit Pont in Paris, *Nouvelles Récréations et joyeux devis* I–XC, ed. Krystyna Kasprzyk (Paris: Honoré Champion, 1980), Nouvelle 63, 233–37. Overwhelmed ("accablé") by the *harangere*, the scholar retreats to the "college de Montaigue."

CHAPTER 3

1. Losse, "Old World Meets the New," 85–100. My article draws on the work of Eamon, "Cannibalism and Contagion," 1–31. Eamon points out that the surgeon Leonardo Fioravanti advanced the theory that the syphilis epidemic in Italy had been caused by the practice of using the dead body parts of soldiers during the French invasion of Naples as a base for food in the soldiers' camps (Eamon, 10, 11). For cannibalism as a violation of natural law, see also Pagden, *The Fall of Natural Man*, 80–87.

2. Thevet, *Histoire d'André Thevet Angoumoisin*, 211.

3. Janet Whatley, in her translation of Léry's work, *History of a Voyage to the Land of Brazil*, notes the separate origins of yaws and syphilis. Yaws is rooted in the *treponema pertenue* and not the *treponema pallida*, the source of syphilis, but Francesco Guerra points out in his article, noted in the following, that these two strains are morphologically indistinguishable. In another article, "The Origins of Syphilis," Harrison comments on the attribution of syphilis as the "Great Imitator" (1–7). One of the clearest explanations of the relationships of various types of syphilis is to be found in an article by Guerra, "The Problem of Syphilis," 845–51. Summarizing the work of L. H. Turner, Guerra states that the treponemes of *pinta* (found only in America), yaws (found in the moist and hot climates of central Africa and the East and West Indies), endemic syphilis (found in the hot, arid climates of Northern and Southern Africa, Arabia, Siberia, and central Australia), and venereal syphilis (developed and now existing in urban society) "are morphologically indistinguishable" and progress from an early stage of primary and secondary lesions to a latent stage ending with tertiary lesions (846).

4. Léry, *Histoire d'un voyage*, 109. All citations in English follow the translation of Janet Whatley in *History of a Voyage to the Land of Brazil*, 4. In his book *Le Huguenot et le sauvage* (Geneva: Droz, 2004), Frank Lestringant surmises that Léry's decision to publish his memoirs of his travel to Brazil served both his own and his Huguenot party's purpose: "On comprend donc comment l'*Histoire* de Léry réalise la synthèse entre un projet littéraire personnel et la commande passée par les représentants du parti Huguenot" (97; translation mine) [So we come to understand just how much de Léry's *History* brings about the synthesis between an individual literary enterprise and a charge past through the officials of the Huguenot party].

5. Fernel d'Amiens, *Le Meilleur traitement du Mal Vénérien*, 27.

6. Harrison worked with Dr. A. Cavaillon, president of the International Union against Venereal Disease, to confirm the dates of the earliest mention of urban edicts in France demanding that individuals infected with "la grosse vérole" leave the confines of the city in question (Harrison, "The Origins of Syphilis," 6.

7. Anatole de Montaiglon includes this poem in a volume of poetry extending from the reign of Louis XII (1498–1515) to the end of the Valois line, at the death of Henri III in 1589. He goes on to note that these for the most part anonymous works reveal what is on the mind of the people: "Tout ce qui a occupé ces époques, tout ce qui les caractérise, s'y trouve représenté; les idées religieuses, les satires catholiques ou protestantes;—l'histoire, la petite encore plus que la grande, par les pieces de circonstance" *Recueil de poésies françoises des XVe et XVIe siècles: morales, facétieuses, historiques*, ed. Anatole de Montaiglon, 3 vols. (Paris: P. Jannet, 1855), I: 68–72; I: vii. For more on the Evangelical humanist writers' satirical use of Latin in an irreverent context to satirize the abuses and shortcomings of the Catholic clergy, see Deborah N. Losse, "Parler le latin de leur mere. Code-Switching: Latinisms to Mark Satirical Intent in the Renaissance Tale," *La Satire dans tous ses états*, ed. Bernd Renner (Geneva: Droz, 2009), 92–103.

8. In "Erasmus' Prescription for Henry VIII," Boyle cites heavily from a letter addressed by Erasmus to Henry VIII of England, in which the former dedicates his *Paraphrasis in evangelium Lucae* to King Henry VIII and argues "the therapeutic and preservative powers of the gospel" (167). She references *Erasmi epistolae*, ed. P. S. Allen et al., 12 vols. (Oxford: Oxford University Press, 1906–53), V: 1313–1322. See Persels, "The Sorbonnic Trots," 1089–1111. He evokes the opposition of the perverted Satanus medicus and the sovereign Christus medicus in his treatment of the Calvinist Conrad Badius's *Comédie du pape malade et tirant à la fin* (1561), 1108.

9. Arbesmann, "The Concept of 'Christus Medicus' in St. Augustine," 1–28. In *The Renaissance Hospital*, Henderson notes the "awareness" of the Augustinian concept of Christus medicus in Renaissance Florence. An image of Christ touching a wound in his side, "as depicted in Bicci di Lorenzo's fresco," is placed as a lunette over the doorway leading to the cemetery of the Hospital of Santa Maria Nuova (114–15). Henderson mentions as well a familiarity with the thirteenth-century Dominican friar Domenico Cavalca, whose work *Lo specchio della croce* reports that Christ "came as a doctor not just to visit us, but to cure us" (115).

10. Rabelais, *Pantagruel*, in *Oeuvres completes*, 215; Rabelais, *Complete Works*, 134. All quotations with the exception of note 9 will be from *Oeuvres completes* and translations from the English translation, *The Complete Works of François Rabelais*.

11. See Bakhtin, *L'Oeuvre de François Rabelais*, 164, 175. See also the English translation, Bakhtin, *Rabelais and His World*, 161, 173. "La goutte et la vérole "joyeuses maladies," resultant d'un abus immoderé de *nourriture, boisson et plaisirs sexuels,* sont par consequent substantiellement liées au 'bas' materiel et corporel. La vérole était encore à l'époque la 'maladie à la mode,' alors que le theme de la goutte était déjà répandu dans le réalisme grotesque" (164/161) [Gout and syphilis are "gay diseases," the result of overindulgence in food, drink, and sexual intercourse. They are essentially connected with the material bodily lower stratum. Pox was still a "fashionable disease" in those days. As to gout, it was widespread in grotesque realism].

12. Montaiglon, "Les Sept marchans de Naples," II: 99–111; n. 1, 99: "Marchans n'a pas ici son sens le plus ordinaire de vendeur, mais, au contraire, celui d'acheteur."

13. Noël du Fail, *Propos rustiques,* ed. Gabriel-André Pérouse and Roger Dubuis (Geneva: Droz, 1994), 97. The depiction of Tailleboudin with his games brings to mind the depiction of Panurge as a prankster and perpetual youth, always taking advantage of those gullible enough to believe in indulgences and those whose self-righteous attitude makes them ready targets for clever, street-wise adolescents (*Pantagruel*, ch. 16)

14. Pérouse and Dubois note in their introduction that Noël du Fail seems to have been a supporter of the reform movement during one period, but other evidence suggests that he was "bel et bien catholique" (8). I recognize that he was indeed eager to reform the church and its abuses: indulgences, pilgrimages, and undue belief in the power of the saints to intervene in stopping the advance of medical infirmities. In short, his seems to be a belief in the power of the individual to appeal directly to God. In evoking the "gros chanoine" who takes up with the young woman, he attacks the hypocrisy of the clergy. Dominique Bertrand comments on the "tensions sensibles" between the appeal to oral tradition in Du Fail and the traces of the "savant humaniste" in his work. There exists, she points out, a heterogeneity of style in his tales, especially in the evolution between the *Propos rustiques* and the *Balivernies, ou Contes nouveaux d'Eutrapel, autrement dit Léon Ladulphy.* The fact that Du Fail takes up the name of an interlocutor used by Erasmus in the colloquy "The New Mother" or "Puerpera," discussed earlier, reveals his ties to Evangelical humanism. While observing the pull between oral and written styles,

popular and learned contexts, Bertrand acknowledges that Du Fail remains conscious of the difference between the two levels and quotes Marie-Claude Bichard-Thomine's conclusion that he never arrives at the "heureux mélange des langages" that can be found in Rabelais: Dominique Bertrand, "Autrement dire: les jeux du pseudonyme chez Noël du Fail," *Seizième Siècle* 1 (2005): 265–66. Cited by Bertrand, Marie-Claude Bichard-Thomine, *Noël Du Fail, conteur* (Paris: Champion, 2001), XCI.

15. *Satyres chrestiennes de la cuisine papale,* xvi. Citations will be from this edition; translations are mine. Chamay notes the findings of Eugénie Droz in "L'auteur des *Satyres chrestiennes de la cuisine papale,*" in *Les Chemins de l'hérésie* (Geneva: Slatkine, 1976), 4: 81–100. In "Les Satyres chrestiennes de la cuisine papale: Jeux et enjeux d'un texte de combat," in *La Satire dans tous ses états,* ed. Bernd Renner (Geneva: Droz, 2009), 267–84, Chamay and Bernd Renner comment upon the vacillation between the ad hominem attack on Pierre Lizet in this work with the less direct and more nuanced attacks on other Catholic polemicists that is common in the satiric poetry of the period. They do note the particularly vitriolic language of which Lizet is the target (267–84). The acerbic language of the *Satyres chrestiennes de la cuisine papale* is an example, as pointed out by Bernd Renner, of the passage from more playful Horatian satire to the scathing satire characteristic of Juvenal. The latter marks the transition to the violent years of the Wars of Religion. See Renner, "*From* Satura *to* Satyre," 390–91.

16. Frank Lestringant, "Catholiques et cannibales: Le thème du cannibalisme dans le discours protestant du temps des guerres de religion," in *Pratiques et discours alimentaires à la renaissance: Actes du colloque de Tours 1979,* ed. J.-C. Margolin and R. Sauzet (Paris: Maisonneuve et Larose, 1982), 233–45.

17. References will be made to Désiré, *Le contrepoison des cinquante-deux chansons de Clément Marot.* Marot's work (*Cinquante deux psalmes de David. Traduictz en rithme Françoise selon la verité Hebraïque, par Clement Marot. Avec plusieurs autres compositions tant dudict Autheur que d'autres, non jamais encore imprimées* [Paris: Estienne Groulleau, 1549]) was fundamental in making the beauty of the psalms accessible to Evangelical Reform-minded Christians, and Désiré understood the threat to the Catholic Church.

18. G. Wylie Sypher comments: "[the Catholic] insistence upon identifying Protestantism and any toleration of it with moral corruption stemmed from an underlying conviction that the current advance of heresy was *symptomatic* [emphasis mine] of a general moral crisis manifest throughout society" ("'Faisant ce qu'il leur vient à plaisir': The Image of Protestantism in French Catholic Polemic on the Eve of the Religious Wars," *The Sixteenth Century Journal* 111, no. 2 [Summer 1980]: 60). John Henderson mentions the moral component brought to the discussion of diseases in the later sixteenth century by the Counter-Reformation. He states that those admitted after 1574 to the Incurabili hospital in Florence where the pox was treated had to produce both a "certificate from their physician of having need to take the wood [guaiacum] and a certificate from their parish priest that they are really poor and cannot afford to treat themselves" (110). The Incurabili hospitals were set up specifically to deal with "incurable" diseases, and especially the *Mal Francese* or French disease (Henderson, 267).

19. See Katherine Maynard, "'Miel empoisonné': Satire and Sickness in Ronsard's *Discours des misères de ce temps,*" in *La Satire dans tous ses états,* ed. Bernd Renner (Geneva: Droz, 2009), 245–64. Maynard states that Ronsard links the Protestants to melancholy by their very unkempt and withdrawn appearance: "le front de rides labouré"; "les cheveux mal peignez" (578, vv. 5–6). Olivier Pot, as Maynard comments, speaks of the "complète médicalisation du problème thólogique" (252), here evoked not in terms

of the pox but in a diagnosis of melancholy (201). See Olivier Pot, "Prophétie et mélancolie. La querelle entre Ronsard et les protestants (1562–65)," *in Prophètes et prophéties au XVI*^{e} *siècle, Cahiers V-L Saulnier* 15 (Paris: Presses de l'ENS, 1998): 189–229.

20. Ronsard, "Continuation du discours des miseres de ce temps," in *Oeuvres complètes*, II: 551.

21. "Response de Pierre de Ronsard aux injures et calomnies de je ne scay quels Prédicantereaux et Ministreaux de Genéve," *Oeuvres complètes*, II: 595–621. See reference to page 597, verse 36, on page 1097. Explaining the reference on page 597, "Qui remonte et repousse aux Enfers un rocher / Dont tu as pris ton nom" [Who in Hell pushes uphill and back down a rock, / A rock whose name you took for your own], Gustave Cohen remarks that hidden in this reference to rock is the real-life model for Brother Zamariel, Antoine de la Roche-Chandieu: "Antoine de La Roche-Chandieu, mais c'est le nom réel de son adversaire Zamariel." (1097).

22. Perhaps to preclude further comparisons between himself and Zamariel, Ronsard suppressed references to his own delight in female conversation and affection after 1573, as civil conflict was accelerating in the wake of massacre of Saint Barthélemy: "J'aime à faire l'amour, j'aime à parler aux femmes," a line that follows "Je ne loge chez moy trop de severité," line 550. See *Oeuvres complètes*, II: 1098, n. 18.

23. Ronsard's appropriation of Reformed rhetorical strategies perhaps confirms François Rigolot's assertion that Ronsard turns civic strife into rhetorical contention. See François Rigolot, "Poétique et politique: Ronsard et Montaigne devant les troubles de leur temps," in *Ronsard et Montaigne: écrivains engagés?*, ed. Michel Dassonville (Lexington, KY: French Forum, 1989), 57–69. See also Szabari, *Less Rightly Said*, 145–46.

24. It is known that Ronsard was keenly aware of Huguenot sensibilities about the lack of public confession in the Catholic Church. In his "Continuation du discours des miseres de ce temps," he critiques Huguenot hypocrisy in insisting on open confession but failing to throw themselves into the process in a sincere and heartfelt manner: "Jesus, que seulement vous confessez ici / De bouche et non de coeur, ne faisoit pas ainsi" (II: 551, vv. 12–13).

25. E. T. Dubedout noted early in the twentieth century that Ronsard's antipathy for Reform theology is rooted as much in his faith in his country as it is in his Catholic beliefs. The two go hand in hand: "La Réforme, odieuse à Ronsard catholique, le fut davantage peut-être à Ronsard patriote," "Le 'Discours' de Ronsard," *Modern Philology* 1, no. 3 (January 1904): 447. Dubedout urges us to see in the "Response" the sincerity of his faith and the ardor of his patriotism (456). To read the poem in the light of civil and religious conflict is to go beyond the role of Ronsard as courtier and to understand the double motivation for writing: his faith and his patriotism. See also Daniel Ménager, *Ronsard: Le roi, le poète et les hommes* (Geneva: Droz, 1979), 167–85, cited in Szabari, *Less Rightly Said*, 139. Szabari states: "Ronsard attributes first and foremost a political and civic function to religion, namely, that it assures the links between people in a society" (252, n. 40).

26. Ullrich Langer, "A Courtier's Problematic Defense: Ronsard's 'Response aux injures,'" *Bibliothèque d'Humanisme et Renaissance* 46, no. 2 (1984): 343–55.

27. Langer notes that it was the last major polemical piece written against the Protestants before the edict of September 1663, forbidding inflammatory texts (Langer, 345, n. 3).

28. D'Aubigné, "De la mort du roi à l'Assemblée de Saumur," in *Oeuvres*, II: 230.

CHAPTER 4

1. See Géralde Nakam's edition of Jean de Léry's *Histoire mémorable du siège de Sancerre,* 292: Léry, *Au lendemain de la Saint-Barthélemy. Guerre civile et famine. Histoire mémorable du siège de Sancerre de Jean de Léry,* ed. Géralde Nakam (Paris: Éditions Anthropos, 1975). To make a distinction between Nakam's lengthy and detailed introduction and Léry's original text, reference will be made to *Au lendemain de la Saint-Barthélemy* when Nakam's introduction is concerned and to *Histoire mémorable du siège de Sancerre* when Léry's text is cited. Léry speaks of the "appetit desordonné" of the husband, wife, and old lady who were caught consuming the limbs and parts of their three-year-old daughter who had died of hunger during the siege of Sancerre.

2. "Sur Jean de Léry. Entretien avec Claude Lévi-Strauss. Propos recueillis par Dominique-Antoine Grisoni," in Léry, *Histoire d'un voyage,* 7. In his interview, Claude Lévi-Strauss reveals the similarities between his own life and that of Jean de Léry: the age at which they composed their work on the indigenous peoples of Brazil, the time elapsed between the stay in Brazil and the final redaction and publication of their work, and the wars (Wars of Religion for Léry, World War II for Lévi-Strauss) and subsequent persecution brought on by the wars that they witnessed.

3. Brazilwood ink was red in substance and made from a liquid extract of brazilwood. Lestringant reports that it was also used for dying cloth (*Histoire d'un voyage,* 61, n. 1). All quotations from the French will refer to the fine edition of Frank Lestringant, and English translations will be those of Janet Whatley's very readable translation of Léry's work, *History of a Voyage to the Land of Brazil,* xlv.

4. Montaigne, *Les Essais,* "Des Cannibales" I: 31, 209; *The Complete Essays of Montaigne,* 155. All references to the *Essais* will be to this first edition; translations will reference *The Complete Essays*. See also my essay, "Rewriting Culture: Montaigne Recounts New World Ethnography," *Neophilologus* 83 (1999): 517–28.

5. Frank Lestringant describes this type of cannibalism as "le cannibalisme de vengeance" [cannibalism of vengeance], where descriptions appear of the vicious repression carried out by Catholics against Huguenots and where in the massacre of Saint-Barthélemy, Catholics are described by Protestants as eating the livers and hearts of massacred Huguenots ("Catholiques et cannibales," 233–45). Lestringant describes initially four types of cannibalism present in the Protestant polemical writings: cannibalism of vengeance (*cannibalisme de vengeance*); habitual cannibalism (*cannibalisme de coutume*), such as one finds in maritime folklore of starving sailors; cannibalism of hunger (*cannibalisme de famine*), found in stories of siege or famine; and criminal cannibalism (*cannibalisme criminel*), in which an individual will punish another for betrayal by feeding him or her parts of a human being. In the end, Lestringant states that these four constitute two categories of cannibalism: forced cannibalism (*cannibalisme de contrainte*) and violent cannibalism (*cannibalisme de violence;* 233).

6. Andrea Frisch points out that Léry's comparative eye stops short of condoning the nudity of the Tupinamba women. The beauty of the Tupi women could stand up to that of the European woman, but the excesses ("superfluitez") of European clothing were neither more or less praiseworthy ("louables") than Tupi nudity—both lacked modesty. "Léry's espousal of a Calvinist 'modesty' creates a standard according to which both Europeans and Americans fall short," "In a Sacramental Mode: Jean de Léry's Calvinist Ethnography," *Representations* 77, no. 1 (Winter 2002): 88. Frisch notes that his

Calvinist antipathy for resemblance, most evident in the Catholic belief in the transformation of the Host into the body of Christ, the wine into the blood of Christ, leads Léry to note differences, as in the contrast of the nudity of the Tupinamba women and the exaggerated finery of the Europeans (91). "In the sacrament of the Lord's Supper, according to Calvin, 'the Spirit is the primary witness who gives us a full assurance of this testament [of the Eucharist].'" Frisch cites the *Institutes of the Christian Religion,* trans. Henry Beveridge (Grand Rapids, MI: Eerdmans, 1957), 597. She also cites the French: "Le Saint-Esprit, qui est le principal témoin, nous prouve avec certitude ce témoignage, nous le fait croire, entendre et reconnaître; car autrement nous ne le pourrions comprendre," *Institution de la religion chrétienne, Institutio christianae religionis* (Geneva, 1955), 4.14.22. 288. This translation is based on the 1560 French edition of Calvin's work. See also Andrea Frisch, *The Invention of the Eye Witness: Witnessing and Testimony in Early Modern France* (Chapel Hill: North Carolina Studies in Romance Languages and Literatures #29, 2004), 161.

7. Lestringant notes the polemical nature of accusations of "paillardise," especially in the rhetoric between Catholics and Protestants (*Histoire d'un voyage,* 181, n. 1). I would add that in the sixteenth century, after the first outbreak of syphilis on the return of Columbus's sailors to Europe and the rapid spread among the French, Spanish, Italian, Swiss and other European soldiers in Italy, the consequences of "paillardise" took on disastrous dimensions.

8. In his *Histoire des deux voyages* (1587–88), yet another rendering of his travel, Thevet speaks of the "maladie des Pians" and correctly attributes the cause to sexual transmission during intercourse. Having commented that the Tupinamba are close to animals by nature and given to lechery ("Car ce peuple, comme il est brutal, est fort addonné à la paillardise"), Thevet blames the libidinous inclinations of women: "Qui me fait penser . . . que de cette malversation, et compagnie avec ces femmes ainsy eschuaffées, cette maladie a pris sa source, et n'est autre chose que cette belle verole": Thevet, *Histoire d'André Thevet,* 211. I am reminded of Thevet's Franciscan education and the powerful influence of the teachings of Saint Paul about the sexual appetites of women. Rabelais's *Tiers Livre* and his portrait of the theologian Hippothadée and the physician Rondibilis (chapters 30–33) come to mind: Rabelais, *Oeuvres complètes,* 478–94. In regards to *pians,* it is often translated as "yaws," rooted in the *treponema pertenue,* as compared to the source of syphilis, from the *treponema pallida.* In his article "The Problem of Syphilis," Francesco Guerra notes that the two strains are morphologically indistinguishable.

9. *Dix Livres de la Chirurgie, avec Le Magasin des Instrumens necessaires à icelle,* (Paris: Jean le Royer, 1564). Rpt. Paris: Cercle du Livre Précieux, n.d.

10. Fernel d'Amiens, *Le Meilleur traitement du Mal Vénérien,* 27.

11. William Eamon discusses one of the most notorious surgeons who treated syphilis, Leonardo Fioravanti, and his theory that the disease, in the Old World and the New, came from eating one's own kind. Running counter to the more established belief that syphilis was a new disease imported to the Old World by Columbus's sailors on their return to Europe, he attributes the disease to the army cooks during the French invasion of Italy in the last decade of the fifteenth century. He cites their practice of making stews out of dead soldiers as the source of syphilis. He says that the cooks would "secretly take the flesh from the bodies of the dead and use it to make certain dishes." Leonardo Fioravanti, *Capricci medicinali dell'eccelente medico & cirurgico M. Leonardo Fioravanti, Bolognese. Divisi in Tre Libri, col privilegio.* In Venezia, Ludovico Avanzo, 1561, 49v, cited by Eamon, "Cannibalism and Contagion," 10–11. He also credits Pagden: "As

Anthony Pagden has pointed out, this view [that men who ate other men must be subhuman] was premised upon an understanding of cannibalism as a violation of the natural law forbidding the eating of one's own kind" (Eamon 18): Pagden, *The Fall of Natural Man*, 80–89.

12. In his preface to the *Histoire d'un voyage,* Léry maintains:

> Mais quant en ceste presente année de 1577, lisant la Cosmographie de Thevet, j'ay veu que il n'a pas seulement renouvelé et augmenté ses premiers erreurs, mais, qui plus est . . . sans autre occasion, que l'envie qu'il a euë de mesdire et detracter des Ministres, et par consequent de ceux qui en l'an 1556, les accompanerent pour aller trouver Villegagnon en la terre du Bresil, dont j'estois du nombre, avec des digressions fausses, piquantes, et injurieuses, nous a imposé des crimes; à fin, di-je, de repousser ces impostures de Thevet, j'ay esté comme contraint de mettre en lumiere to le discours de nostre voyage. (63/xlvi)

> But in this present year 1577, reading Thevet's *Cosmography*, I saw that he has not only revived and augmented his early errors, but what is more . . . , with no other pretext than the desire to backbite and, with false, stinging, and abusive digressions, to slander the ministers and those—of whom I was one—who in 1556 accompanied them to go join Villegagnon in Brazil, he has imputes to us crimes. Therefore, in order to refute these falsehoods of Thevet, I have been compelled to set forth a complete report of our voyage.

13. In her article, "'And the Word became Flesh . . .': Cannibalism and Religious Polemic in the Poetry of Desportes and d'Aubigné," *Renaissance and Reformation/ Renaissance et Réforme* 24, no. 1 (2000): 45–56, Susan K. Silver remarks on d'Aubigné's tendency, "offset by an antithesis an absolute evil in order to foreground an exemplary good" (50). Léry engages in the same contrast—of cannibalism by nonbelievers or papists as opposed to the strength of the Huguenots to withstand the horrors of famine and whatever cruel means of persecution may be meted out by the Catholic cause.

14. Gérallde Nakam states: "Notre auteur a été interlocuteur privilégié et le protégé de La Châtre et de Sarrieu" (Léry, *Histoire mémorable du siège de Sancerre,* 111) [Our author was a privileged interlocutor and protégé of La Châtre and Sarrieu]. She goes on to speculate that the Catholic leadership preferred Léry over Johanneau, who was already marked by his two rebellions against Catholic forces., but she admits that a legend had developed around Léry's personality because of his time in Brazil (111–12).

15. "Après Érasme et avant Montaigne, usant comme eux du paradoxe, Léry engage fermement à se méfier des apparences et du 'cuyder' présomptueux" (*Au lendemain de la Saint-Barthélemy*, 83).

16. See Frisch, "In a Sacramental Mode," 95: "Léry's appeal to his own discourse locates both the authority and the referent of his testimony in the eternal present of his text." Since the *Histoire mémorable du siège de Sancerre* was written first, it is likely that the technique of self-citation was begun in this work and then resumed by Léry when he wrote the definitive version of the *Histoire d'un voyage faict en la terre de Brésil.*

17. "Mais, ô Dieu eternel! voicy encores le comble de toute misere et du jugement de Dieu. Car comme il proteste en sa Loy qu'il reduira ceux qui n'obeiront à ses Commandemends en tel estat, que durant le siege il fera que les meres mangeront leurs enfans" (*Histoire mémorable du siège de Sancerre,* 290) [But o eternal God, here is again the

height of all misery and Divine Judgment. For as he proclaims in his Law (The Book of Deuteronomy) that he will reduce those who do not obey his Commandments to such a state that during the siege he will have the mothers eat their children]. See also *Histoire d'un voyage faict en la terre du Brésil,* 535, n. 2. Léry explains earlier in this same chapter of the *Histoire d'un voyage faict en la terre du Brésil* that the hunger during the siege of Sancerre was not as bad as that they experienced on board ship on the return voyage to Europe. In Sancerre they had water and wine, herbs and vine shoots (533/211). This is another example of self-citation—the moving backwards and forwards from the first *Histoire* to the second. It allows Léry to point out once again that the famine in Sancerre was one of the most difficult that he had ever heard about. The subtext is also that the famine was caused by the cruelty of one sect persecuting another—one sect trying to wipe out those enlightened by the Reformation.

18. In comparing cannibalism in the New World to excessive cruelty in the Old, Léry will recycle the phrase "succer le sang et la moëlle" to speak of usurers sucking the blood of widows, orphans, and the poor and eating them alive (*Histoire d'un voyage en la terre du Brésil,* 375/132), cited earlier in this chapter.

CHAPTER 5

1. Eamon, "Cannibalism and Contagion," 5.
2. Eamon credits Oviedo as the first to mention that the crew of Columbus became infected after relations with the indigenous people in the New World and brought the disease to Europe on their return (6). See, as cited by Eamon, Gonzalo Fernández de Oviedo y Valdes, *Historia general y natural de las Indias,* I: 55. See also Bartolomé de las Casas, *Historia de las Indias,* 5 vols. (Madrid, 1876), 5: 349 and Richard Holcomb, "Ruy Diaz de Isla and the Haitian Myth of European Syphilis," *Medical Life* 45 (1956): 270–315.
3. Montaigne, *Les Essais,* II: 37, 772; *Complete Essays,* 586. All quotations from the French text refer to the first source; all translations from the *Essais* refer to *Complete Essays.* It is customary to acknowledge the changes/additions made by Montaigne by referring to the particular editions in which the text appears: 1580 or A, 1588 or B, and to C, the revisions made on the Bordeaux copy in the hand of the author subsequent to the publication of the edition of 1588 up to Montaigne's death in 1592.
4. Antonia Szabari, "'parler seulement de moy': The Disposition of the Subject in Montaigne's Essay 'De l'art de conferer,'" *MLN* 116, no. 5 (December 2001): 1001–24.
5. For a discussion of whether syphilis was a new disease imported from the New World or an ancient disease, see Claude Quétel, *The History of Syphilis,* trans. Judith Braddock and Brian Pike (Baltimore: Johns Hopkins University Press, 1992), 34–40.
6. Eamon, 18. See Pagden, *The Fall of Natural Man,* 80–87.
7. Losse, "Rewriting Culture," 517–28.
8. Dudley D. Marchi, "Montaigne and the New World: The Cannibalism of Cultural Production," *Modern Language Studies* 23, no. 4 (Autumn 1993): 37.
9. Fioravanti, *Capricci medicinali,* 237v–238. An earlier work makes the same point about expelling the flatterers and restoring order to the body politic: *Delle speccho di scientie universale* (Venice, 1572), 140–45. Both works are cited by Eamon, 20.
10. Eamon, 22. Leonardo Fioravanti, *Della fisica* (Venice, 1582), 302.
11. Mary Douglas, *Natural Symbols: Explorations in Cosmology* (New York: Vintage Books, 1973), 93; cited by Eamon, 21.
12. In *Inventing the Indigenous: Local Knowledge and Natural History in Early*

Modern Europe (Cambridge: Cambridge University Press, 2007), Alix Cooper explains the tendency of Paracelsus and other medical humanists to favor local remedies rather than expensive drugs or herbs brought from exotic places (30). She cites Charles Webster, "Paracelsus: Medicine as Popular Protest, " in *Medicine and the Reformation,* ed. Ole Peter Grell and Andrew Cunningham (London: Routledge, 1993), 70. Cooper highlights several trends in sixteenth-century medicine. First, she mentions the preference for "simples" from "plant, animal, and mineral sources," favored by the newly edited Greek editions of ancient medical texts over compound medicines, touted by Arabic medical practices and appropriated by medieval apothecaries (Cooper, 29). Second, she describes the rise of a certain medical nationalism that came from the call for local medicines begun in Germany by Paracelsus in the 1520s and continued by Symphorien Champier in France in 1533, as evidenced in his *Hortus Gallicus, pro Gallis in Gallia scriptus* or *French Garden, Written for the French in France* (Lyon, in aedibus Melchioris et Gasparis Trechsel fratrum, 1533) (Cooper, 36). Finally, she refers to the spilling over of Catholic/Protestant tensions into medicine. In his *Herbarius,* Paracelsus touts the superior quality of German medicine, previously hidden by the mean-spirited and ignorant Italians: "Indeed these medicines [those of German origin] are so good that neither Italy, France, nor any other realm can boast of better ones. That this has not come to light for such a long time is the fault of Italy, the mother of ignorance and inexperience": "The *Herbarius* of Paracelsus," ed. Bruce Moran, *Pharmacy in History* 35 (1993): 104, and Paracelsus, "Herbarius Theophrasti de virtutibus herbarum, radicum seminum etc Alemaniae, patriae et imperII," in Theophrast von Hohenheim gen. *Paracelsus Sämtliche Werke. I. Abteilung: Medizinische, naturwissenschaftliche und philosophiche Schriften,* ed. Karl Sudhoff (Munich & Berlin: Oldenbourg, 1930), 2: 3; cited by Cooper, 27. It is clear that the medical debate of the sixteenth century reflects the tensions between countries and between religions.

13. Jean Starobinski, "The Body's Moment," *Yale French Studies* 64 (1983): 273–305. Starobinski notes the similarities between the writings of Ambroise Paré and the statement by Montaigne that old age is a type of sickness (280): "La vieillesse, quelque gaillarde qu'elle soit, est de sa nature *comme une espece de maladie*"; Ambroise Paré, *Les Oeuvres,* "Premier livre de l'introduction à la chirurgie," ch. 17. Starobinski quotes from the eighth edition (Paris, 1628), 29.

14. Cited by Cooper, 36. Symphorien Champier, *Hortus gallicus, pro Gallis in Gallia scriptus* (Lyon: in aedibus Melchioris et Gasparis Trechsel fratrum, 1533).

15. Having criticized the disruptive medical practices of contemporary physicians, the essayist feels compelled to give a long justification for why he engages in thermal treatments. In spite of the fact that he hasn't noticed any extraordinary or miraculous benefits to his health ("aucun effect extraordinarie et miraculeux," II: 37, 776A/590), he finds that the water is not unpleasant to the taste nor harmful, just a natural and simple treatment: "elle est naturelle et simple, qui aumoins n'est pas dangereuse"; 776A/590). See also Deborah N. Losse, *Montaigne and Brief Narrative Form: Shaping the Essay* (Basingstoke: Palgrave Macmillan, 2013), 149. In a witty and informative article, Tom Conley traces the evolution of Michel de Montaigne's "dispathie naturelle à la medecine" back to his family heritage and follows the graphic association of the family ailment, *pierre,* to the given name of Montaigne's father (*père*) Pierre, "From Antidote to Anecdote: Montaigne on Dissemblance," *SubStance* 38, no. 1, issue 118: The Anecdote (2009): 5–15.

16. Cooper, 36; Champier, 7–8.

17. Gérald Nakam, *Montaigne et son temps: Les événement et les Essais. L'Histoire, la vie et le livre* (Paris: A.-G. Nizet, 1982), 198.

18. Working in the southwest of France and in the same decade as Montaigne, Jacques Auguste de Thou, composing his *Hieracosophion,* or treatise on falconry, uses the word "pestilence" to describe the decline in military discipline and absence of respect for the law during the disruptions brought on by the Wars of Religion: "Cette pestilence se répand imperceptiblement et s'insinue jusque dans les esprits des nobles"; Ingrid A. R. De Smet, *La Fauconnerie à la Renaissance. Le Hierocosophion (1582–84) de Jacques Auguste de Thou,* édition critique, traduction et commentaire précédés d'une étude historique de la chasse au vol en France au XVIe siècle (Geneva: Librairie Droz, 2013), 276–77. The reference to the progression of the disease through the body as it ultimately attacks the brain recalls the passage of syphilis through the body. As Montaigne will do, de Thou denounces the displacement of old values ("les excellents arts de la paix, par lesquels nous vivons" [Quinetiam eximiae pacis, queis vivimus, artes]) to engage in civil war: "attaquer, piller et vaguer impunément" [Grassari et praedas agere, atque impune vagari] ("Premier Livre," vv. 837–38, 276–77). He too is upset by the lack of respect for the law. He comments that the enormous waste of human and material resources in the civil wars has depleted the moral and physical fiber of France (276–77). It is of significant interest that the first edition of the *Hieracosophion* was published in Bordeaux by Simon Millanges, Montaigne's first publisher, just two years after the publication of the first edition of the *Essais.* As Brenton Hobart observes in his recently defended dissertation directed by Frank Lestringant, war has long been linked to pestilence, as can be seen in the works of Homer, Thucydides, and Virgil, among others. Hobart shows how Paré, in his *Traicté de la peste, de la petite verolle & rougeolle: avec une brefve description de la lepre* (1568), appropriates the image of the plague with all its ravages to describe the corruption that rages through the many provinces that make up France, torn apart by the civil wars. See Brenton Hobart, "L'imaginaire de la peste dans la littérature française de la Renaissance" (Thèse pour obtenir le grade de Docteur de l'Université Paris-Sorbonne, 8 janvier 2014), 332. As Fioravanti and Montaigne do, Paré makes the connection between the human body and the body politic, and argues that it is the well-balanced life that preserves the human body as well as the state: "La vie équilibrée, qui permet la préservation du corps humain, sert également à celle du plus grand corps public" (Hobart, 364).

19. Both noted physicians, Fernel and Scaliger died in 1588—around the time of the publication of Montaigne's third book of essays. See III: 13, 1087, n. 16. Changing theories of medicine and changing interpretations of the iterative celebration of the Eucharist destabilized the habits and ritual of Montaigne's life and those of his community. In this regard, Lestringant follows in the *Journal de Vogage* the extensive efforts which Montaigne devoted to seeking out a multitude of Protestant theories on the Eucharist. He interviewed many pastors but was frustrated by the dogmatism and diversity of views. Lestringant suggests that in choosing Catholicism for his personal profession of faith—a religion that had for centuries fortified the kingdom of France—the essayist held to a more moderate view of the Eucharist, one in which the body of Christ is present at certain defined rituals but not at all times and places, as the Lutherans believed, or infrequently and remotely, as the Calvinists held: Lestringant, *Une sainte horreur ou le voyage en eucharistie,* 2nd ed. (Geneva: Droz, 2012), 305–8.

20. Starobinski, 280. Paré, *Les Oeuvres,* 29.

21. Paré, 29, cited by Starobinski, 282–83.

22. Less than thirty years earlier, when the Wars of Religion were heating up, Ronsard applied the same adjective, "monstrueuse," as he addressed his colleague Pierre de Paschal, *historiographe du roi,* "O toy, historien, qui d'encre non menteuse / Escris de

nostre temps l'histoire *monstrueuse,* / Raconte à nos enfans tout ce malheur fatal, / Afin qu'en te lisant ils pleurent nostre mal" ("Discours des misères de ce temps," *Oeuvres complètes,* II: 547, vv. 3–6).

23. Alfred W. Crosby Jr., "The Early History of Syphilis: A Reappraisal," *American Anthropologist,* New Series 71, no. 2 (April 1969): 218–27.

24. Cited by Crosby, 220. Ulrich von Hutten, *Of the Wood Called Guaiacum* (London: Thomas Bertheletreglii, 1540), 2–2r.

25. Cited by Crosby, 218. Von Hutten, *Of the Wood Called Guaiacum,* 1.

26. D'Aubigné, *Oeuvres,* II: 196.

CHAPTER 6

1. See Désiré, *Le contrepoison des cinquante-deux chansons e Clément Marot,* Chanson XXVI, 40, and Montaigne, *Les Essais,* III: 12, 1046. Denis Crouzet's monumental study, *La Nuit de la Saint-Barthélemy,* first published by Fayard in 1994, cites Henri Lancelot Voisin de La Popeleinière, who blamed the corrupted morals of the Huguenot soldiers ("pires qu'Athées et Cannibales" [worse than atheists and cannibals]) for the divine scourge brought down on their people; see Crouzet, 113; Henri Lancelot Voisin de la Popelinière, *L'Histoire de France, enrichie des plus notable occurrances survenues ez provinces de l'Europe et pays voisins, depuis l'an 1550, jusques à ces temps,* par Abraham H, t. II, s.i., 1581, Fol. La21 15, p. 100; Crouzet, 586, n. 4.

2. Kathleen Perry Long comments that every major edict of peace enjoined "oubliance," or "deliberate forgetting of events" and glossing over of suffering; "'Child in the Water': The Spectacle of Violence in Théodore Agrippa d'Aubigné's *Les Tragiques,*" *Dalhousie French Studies* 8 (Winter 2007): 155–65. Long speaks of the imposition of silence in the working of the peace edicts, beginning with the Peace of Amboise (1563), ending the first religious war, and continuing through the Edicts of Boulogne (1573), Beaulieu (1576), and Bergerac (1577) and finally, the Edict of Nantes (1598) (155–56). In *Une sainte horreur,* Lestringant addresses d'Aubigné's expression of his own inability to avenge the suffering of previous generations: "Il sent profondément en lui l'impuissance commune à l'époque, cette faiblesse inhérente à une génération de fils collectivement indignes de succéder à leurs pères" (80) [He felt deeply within himself the impotence of the times, the inner weakness of a generation of sons collectively unworthy of replacing their fathers].

3. See Persels, "The Sorbonnic Trots," 1089–1111.

4. Showing how the Huguenot Jean de Léry, in his *Histoire d'un voyage faict en la terre du Brésil,* internalizes the essential aspects of spiritual witnessing to his own act of testimony as an ethnographer, Frisch underscores how witnessing and testimony become central to Huguenot writing ("In a Sacramental Mode," 82–106). See also Frisch, *Invention of the Eyewitness,* where she demonstrates the legal applications and its extension to narrative. Denis Crouzet also underscores the testimonial function of the Huguenots in attempting to piece together the events of the Saint-Barthélemy massacre, especially for those who had not been in Paris to witness the events (112). The Calvinist historian Simon Goulart writes, in Crouzet's assessment, for those "qui n'ont pas 'veu'" [who had not 'seen'] the massacre (112). A second motivation was to spread the true doctrine and the truth of the events to counteract the lies promulgated by the Catholics. If it was in the best interest of the Catholic royalists to depict their role as forgiving in the light of what they perceived as Protestant plots against the royal family and the Guise family,

then it was incumbent upon the Huguenots to bring together the bits and pieces of the "mémoire collective" of the survivors.

5. D'Aubigné, "Misères," *Les Tragiques*, 268, v. 103; v. 107. It is useful to review Fanlo's notes regarding the dating of the composition of *Les Tragiques*. He designates three periods for the composition: the beginning of Henri III's reign, the period after the conversion of Henri de Navarre to become Henri IV, and the last period after the death of Henri IV (116).

6. Dominick LaCapra, *History and Memory After Auschwitz* (Ithaca: Cornell University Press, 1998), 20.

7. Brenton Hobart shows just how Montaigne's experience of the plague as he and his family were forced to flee is a kind of *dénouement* for the *Essais*. He experienced the physical and moral debilitation caused by the disease itself and the figurative disease—the moral infection wrought by the religious and civil unrest of his times: "Il permet d'enterrer l'ancien Montaigne pour que puisse naître un Montaigne nouveau. Au lieu de s'appuyer sur ses connaissances, il se fie désormais à l'expérience, aux choses vues (dénouement des *Essais* en général)" (420) [This allows the former Montaigne to be buried so that the new Montaigne can be brought to life. Instead of depending on his knowledge, he sets his trust in the experience of things he has witnessed (the conclusion of the *Essais* as a whole)].

8. Léry, *Histoire mémorable du siège de Sancerre (1573) de Jean de Léry*, 327.

9. See also Hobart's description of France's starving and plague-ridden body (438). Lestringant notes that d'Aubigné addresses the way in which the Calvinists viewed the ingestion of the host. Rejecting the theory of transubstantiation and holding to the fact that the bodily sacrifice of Jesus Christ is a unique event that occurred at the time of the Passion, the Calvinists refuse to partake in the cannibalistic act of eating the body of Christ. As seen in "Jugement" of the *Tragiques*, the Huguenots fail to digest a body that cannot be that of Christ and vomit it up as impure, whereas the Catholics participate in the blasphemous act and risk digesting the host and eliminating it through the natural process: "Alors que les catholiques s'exposent au risque d'évacuer Dieu par voies naturelles, les protestants vomissent une chair qui ne peut être Dieu" (85).

10. "Les reîtres, mercenaires allemands vêtus d'un manteau noir, ont été recrutés surtout par les protestants (bien qu'il y en eût aussi dans les armées royales)" (*Les Tragiques*, 284, n. 372) [The reisters, German mercenaries clothed in black coats, were recruited in particular by the Protestants although there were some in the royal armies].

11. Léry mentions "les deux cuisses, jambes et pieds dans une chaudiere de vinaigre, espices et sel, prest à cuire" (*Histoire mémorable du siège de Sancerre*, 291) 'two thighs, legs and feet in a pot with vinegar, spices and salt, ready to cook]. The real cannibalism of the mercenaries, fighting for the radical Catholic cause, mirrors the symbolic cannibalism of the Catholic Mass, where the bread and wine are converted to the body and blood of the Lord—the "sainte horreur," as viewed by the Protestants for whom the sacrifice of Jesus Christ in the passion and resurrection was a unique event and one that could not be repeated at every celebration of the Eucharist: "La christologie de Calvin et de ses disciples insiste par conséquent sur l'unicité de l'incarnation dans son aspect à la fois temporel, le sacrifice de la croix, et spatial, la présence au ciel" (Lestringant, *Une sainte horreur*, 53). Here Lestringant cites Bernard Cottret, *Calvin: Biographie* (Paris: Jean-Claude Lattès, 1995), 273. The mercenary soldiers indulge in exogenic cannibalism—the consumption of human flesh outside of the family. The horror of obsidional cannibalism imposed on the starving population (usually Protestant) of the besieged cities is that

famine drives the people to endogenic cannibalism—the consumption of the flesh of their own family members, their own clan (*Une sainte horreur,* 97).

12. In condemning the Potard family for eating their baby daughter, where the gnawed ears provide evidence of intentional if misguided cannibalism, Léry speaks of "un appetit desordonné" (which I have translated as "wild appetites"), a fact that leads him to comment on "cest cruauté barbare et plus que bestiale" (*Histoire mémorable du siège de Sancerre,* 292) [this savage and more than bestial cruelty].

13. Nakam, *Montaigne et son temps,* 103–4.

14. In "Catholiques et cannibales," Lestringant refers to d'Aubigné's evocation of the escalating cannibalistic fever brought on by the persecution of Huguenots and by the violence of the religious wars (237). In *Une sainte horreur,* Lestringant reinforces d'Aubigné's observation that the mythological figure of Thyeste was duped by Atrée into eating his children. It was not a conscious act of cannibalism. For the families of the besieged, consuming the flesh of their children was a deliberate action brought on by the starvation unleashed by the troops loyal to the Catholic extremists (195): "Les membres de ce fils sont connus au repas, / Et l'autre [Thyeste] estant desceu ne les connoissoit pas" ("Misères," *Les Tragiques,* I: 292, vv. 247–48). The abomination of endogamic cannibalism brought on by the ravages of the civil and religious wars in France is worse than the crime of Thyeste because it was a deliberate, conscious act.

15. In his critical edition of *Les Tragiques,* Fanlo explains that the target of d'Aubigné's criticism of tyranny is the interference of the Guise family in royal affairs. The author looks ahead to the time when the Guise family will be vanquished and "le sceptre des lis joindra le Navarrois" (294, v. 596, n. 596) [the scepter of the lily flower will be join that of Navarre], when France and Navarre will be united under a single scepter and a single monarch.

16. In the *Histoire mémorable du siège de Sancerre,* Léry suggests that the reason the Potards gave way to cannibalism while the others of Sancerre largely did not was that the Potard couple had secretly been married by the Catholic Church rather than waiting, as the Reformed Church had demanded, to confirm the death of the bride's former husband ("Ils s'allerent espouser à la papauté"; *Histoire mémorable du siège de Sancerre,* 292). In both Léry's and d'Aubigné's works, siege-produced famine brings about a reenactment of New World cannibalism, but devoid of the ritualistic meaning it had acquired within Brazilian culture. The tyranny of the *Ligue* forces the inhabitants to engage in cannibalism. Those who abjure their Protestant faith in order to seek relief from salvation are forced to undergo the cannibalistic act of the Catholic Mass, where, through transubstantiation, the host consumed has been transformed into the body of Jesus Christ (Lestringant, *Une sainte horreur,* 97). The Potard family is twice guilty, once for abjuring their Protestant faith, and second for participating in endogamic cannibalism, what Lestringant refers to as "inceste alimentaire" (97).

17. Fanlo states that some of the Huguenot pamphlets had accused the Cardinal of Lorraine of having committed adultery with his sister-in-law Anne d'Este, wife of his brother François de Guise (316, n. 1001–4). The same language of fornication, adultery, sodomy, and incest is applied to the papacy in the final part of *Les Tragiques* ("Jugements," II: 917, vv. 811–16):

> Voicy donc, Antechrist, l'extraict des faicts et gestes,
> Tes fornications, adulteres, incestes,
> Les pechez où nature est tournee à l'envers,

> La bestialité, les grands bourdeaux ouverts,
> Le tribut exigé, la bulle demandee
> Qui a la sodomie en esté concedee;

The papacy is stained by sins against nature—adultery, incest, sodomy, bestiality, and open brothels, for which money was exchanged for permission to indulge in life's pleasures. Such passages confirm Marie-Madeleine Fragonard's observation that d'Aubigné writes at the crossroads of aesthetic and ideological models and that there is a strong tension between the sacred and the profane: "D'Aubigné apparaît comme un carrefour de modèles esthétiques et idéologiques où s'exerce (entre autres) une forte tension entre religieux et profane" (674). See "Les 'chemins enlacez' des *Tragiques*," *Revue d'Histoire Littéraire de la France*, 92e Année, N° 4 (July–August 1992): 669–78. To the false promises and sins of Rome, the martyrs chose Christ, who suffered for them and gave them his water and his bread that they might have their sins forgiven:

> Qui à ma seiche soif, et à mon aspre faim
> Donnastes de bon coeur vostre eau, et vostre pain:
> Venez race du ciel, venez esleus du pere,
> Vos pechez sont esteints, le juge est vostre frere;
> ("Jugement," *Les Tragiques*, II: 922, vv. 873–76)

Fanlo notes that d'Aubigné refers to the papacy as Antichrist and to a succession of papal vices (*Les Tragiques*, 917, nn. 811–17). The Huguenot martyrs as a chosen people have turned their backs on Rome to embrace "l'Eglise universelle" and God's clemency ("la clémence de Dieu"; v. 832; v. 995).

18. Léry points out that the interpreters were paid back for their wanton activities with the Tupi women and describes one notable "natif de Rouen" whose body and face were covered with the telltale red sores of "une maladie incurable qu'ils nomment *Pians*" (*Histoire d'un voyage faict en la terre du Brésil*, 469).

19. D'Aubigné is not alone in critiquing the excesses of fashion among the courtiers. Jacques-Auguste de Thou, in the first edition of his *Hiercosophion,* published by Simon Millanges in 1582, attacks the aristocratic youth for raiding the royal treasuries of "les grands seigneurs" to pay for their fashionable new styles in clothing—high-heeled shoes ("sabots à hauts talons") and breeches embroidered with dazzling gems ("les hauts-de-chausse . . . brodés de gemmes étincelantes" ("Deuxième Livre," 335–36, vv. 10, 12–13). In the second edition of his *Essais* (1588), Montaigne makes similar charges about the new style of courtly fashion for men: "cette vilaine chaussure qui montre si à descouvert nos membres occultes; ce lourd grossissement de pourpoins . . . ces longues tresses de poil effeminées" ("Des loix sumptuaires," I: 43, 269B/197) [this ugly codpiece that so openly shows our secret parts; . . . that heavy stuffing of doublets . . . those long effeminate tresses]. Composing the first edition of his *Essais* around the same time as de Thou was working on the *editio princeps* of his work on falconry, Montaigne joins with de Thou in seeing that these expenses must be cut in order to maintain the royal treasury: if the kings do it, it will happen in a month, but it must begun at court ("que les Rois commencent à quitter ces despences, ce sera faict en un mois"; I: 43, 269A/197).

20. Denis Crouzet comments on the rhetorical element in Huguenot versions of the Saint-Barthélemy massacre and subsequent violence in which emphasis is placed on choosing a life in God in preference to the corrupt life in this world ruled by the Roman Church: "Et, tout au long des années de tribulations, l'agonie, la mort qui saisit l'homme, demeure une invitation pour les vivants à prendre conscience de ce qu'il y une autre vie à

Dieu que celle dans laquelle les maintient l'Église romaine" (160). To die at the hands of the idolaters shows the commitment of a true disciple of Christ and is preferable to life on earth (161). Lestringant shows how the bruises and blood that cover Serpon's daughter's body both disguise and protect her. Her assailants are repelled, and the wounds reveal her as one who has refused to yield to the Catholic "ordures" or blasphemy. The purity of her faith, the whiteness of her soul, is seen by the heavenly Father but goes unobserved by her earthly torturers (*Une sainte horreur,* 81).

21. D'Aubigné, *Oeuvres,* II: Écrits politiques, 191–200; 224–32.

CONCLUSION

1. See Pineaux's introduction to *Le Contrepoison des cinquante-deux chansons de Clément Marot,* 11: "polémiquant ainsi sans relâche contre la Réforme."

2. Paré, *Oeuvres complètes,* II: 527: "extreme nocturnal pains in the head, shoulders, joints." Frank Lestringant mentions a parallel visual representation of the theological infection depicted by Désiré in the Catholic Richard Verstegan's pictures in *Typus Ecclesiae Catholicae/Typus Heretucae Synegogae et eiusdem proprietates* (1585). Verstegan's *Hereticae Synagogae* illustration shows a sharp-nosed villain whispering into the ears of a nun and a monk, presumably getting them to renounce their vows to give way to their lusty passion ("pour mieux paillarder à leur aise"; *Une sainte horreur,* 194). Verbal and visual propaganda depicted sexual wantonness among Protestant and Catholic clergy alike.

3. "Complainte de messire Pierre Liset sur le trespass de son feu nez," *Satyres chrestiennes de la cuisine papale,* 161–62. Remember from chapter 3 that this work was attributed by Eugénie Droz to Théodore de Bèze, "L'auteur des *Satyres chrestiennes de la cuisine papale,*" in *Les Chemins de l'hérésie* (Geneva: Slatkine, 1976), 4: 81–100.

4. Fernel d'Amiens, *Le Meilleur traitement du Mal Vénérien,* 9–10.

5. "Explication familiere et toutesfois mysterique, de l'excellente lettre qui porte pour tiltre, A nostre trescher fils en Christ, Louys de France tres-chrestien, Gregoire Pape XV etc, par Pere A. de la vraye Société de Jesus" (*Oeuvres,* II: 614–15). Jean-Raymond Fanlo observes that the attribution of this letter to Agrippa d'Aubigné is certain (*Oeuvres,* II: 559). He dates the letter to September 1621, following a papal bull from Gregory XV in the first year of his papacy, in which he extols the efforts of Louis XIII to "debeller lesdits heretiques, & reprimer leurs pernicieux efforts & desseins" (561–65).

6. Théodore de Bèze, *Abraham sacrifiant,* ed. Marguerite Soulié and Jean-Dominique Beaudin (Paris: Honoré Champion, 2006), 92, vv. 109–14.

BIBLIOGRAPHY

Ahmed, Ehsan. "Guillaume Briçonnet, Marguerite de Navarre and the Evangelical Critique of Reason." *Bibliothèque d'Humanisme et Renaissance* 69, no. 3 (2007): 615–25.

Arbesmann, Rudolph. "The Concept of Christus *Medicus* in St. Augustine." *Tradition* 10 (1954): 1–28.

Augustine, Saint. *Confessions*. Translated by Pierre de Labriolle. 2 vols. Paris: Les Belles Lettres, 1994.

———. *Confessions*. Translated by R. S. Pine-Coffin. London: Penguin Books, 1961.

Bakhtin, Mikhail. *L'oeuvre de François Rabelais et la culture populaire au moyen âge et sous la renaissance*. Translated by Andrée Robel. Paris: Gallimard, 1970.

———. *Rabelais and His World*. Translated by Hélène Iswolsky. Cambridge, MA: MIT Press, 1968.

Baudouin, François. "Un manuscrit de François Baudouin dans la librairie de Montaigne." *Bibliothèque d'Humanisme et Renaissance* 75 (2013): 105–11.

Bertrand, Dominique. "Autrement dire: les jeux du pseudonyme chez Noël du Fail." *Seizième Siècle* 1 (2005): 257–66.

Bèze, Théodore. *Abraham sacrifiant*. Edited by Marguerite Soulié and Jean-Dominique Beaudin. Paris: Honoré Champion, 2006.

[Bèze, Théodore?]. *Satyres chrestiennes de la cuisine papale*. Edited by Charles-Antoine Chamay. Geneva: Droz, 2005.

Bichard-Thomine, Marie-Claude. *Noël du Fail, conteur*. Paris: Honoré Champion, 2001.

Bierlaire, Franz. *Les Colloques d'Érasme: réforme des études, réforme des moeurs et réforme de l'Eglise au XVIe siècle*. Paris: Les Belles Lettres, 1978.

———. *Érasme et ses colloques: Le livre d'une vie*. Geneva: Droz, 1977.

Boyle, Marjorie O'Rourke. "Erasmus' Prescription for Henry VIII: Logotherapy." *Renaissance Quarterly* 31, no. 2 (1978): 161–72.

Briçonnet, Guillaume, and Marguerite d'Angoulême. *Correspondance (1521–1524)*. Edited by Christine Martineau and Michel Veissière. 2 vols. Geneva: Droz, 1975 and 1979.

Casas, Bartolomé de las. *Historia de las Indias*. 5 vols. Madrid, 1876.

Chamay, Charles-Antoine, and Bernd Renner. "*Les Satyres chrestiennes de la cuisine papale.* Jeux et enjeux d'un texte de combat." In Renner, *La Satire dans tous ses états,* 267–84.

Champier, Symphorien. *Hortus gallicus, pro Gallis in Gallia scriptus.* Lyon: in aedibus Melchioris et Gasparis Trechsel fratrum, 1533.

Conley, Tom. "From Antidote to Anecdote: Montaigne on Dissemblance." *SubStance* 38, no. 1, issue 118: The Anecdote (2009): 5–15.

Cooper, Alix. *Inventing the Indigenous: Local Knowledge and Natural History in Early Modern Europe.* Cambridge: Cambridge University Press, 2007.

Cornell, Barbara. "Malleable Material, Models of Power: Women in Erasmus's 'Marriage Group' and Civility in Boys." *ELH* 57, no. 2 (Summer 1990): 241–62.

Crawford, Katherine. *The Sexual Culture of the French Renaissance.* Cambridge: Cambridge University Press, 2010.

Crosby, Alfred W. Jr. "The Early History of Syphilis: A Reappraisal." *American Anthropologist,* New Series 71, no. 2 (April 1969): 218–27.

Crouzet, Denis. *La nuit de la Saint-Barthélemy: Un rêve perdu de la Renaissance.* Paris: Pluriel, 2012.

D'Aubigné, Agrippa. *Les Tragiques.* Edited by Jean-Raymond Fanlo. 2 vols. Paris: Honoré Champion, 2003.

———. *Oeuvres* II. *Écrits politiques.* Edited by Jean-Raymond Fanlo. Paris: Honoré Champion, 2007.

Désiré, Artus. *Le contrepoison des cinquante-dix chansons de Clément Marot.* Edited by Jacques Pineaux. Geneva: Droz, 1977.

De Smet, Ingrid A. R. *La Fauconnerie à la Renaissance. Le Hierocosophion (1582–84) de Jacques Auguste de Thou.* Édition critique, traduction et commentaire précédés d' une étude historique de la chasse au vol en France au XVIe siècle. Geneva: Librairie Droz, 2013.

Des Périers, Bonaventure. *Nouvelles Récréations et joyeux devis* I–XC. Edited by Krystyna Kasprzyk. Paris: Honoré Champion, 1980.

Diefendorf, Barbara D. *The Saint Bartholomew's Day Massacre: A Brief History with Documents.* Boston/New York: Bedford/Saint Martin's, 2009.

Douglas, Mary. *Natural Symbols: Explorations in Cosmology.* New York, Vintage Books, 1973.

Droz, Eugénie. "L'auteur des *Satyres chrestiennes de la cuisine papale.*" In *Les Chemins de l'hérésie,* vol. 4, 81–100. Geneva: Slatkine, 1976.

Du Fail, Noël. *Les Balivernies d'Eutrapel.* In *Conteurs du seizième siècle.* Edited by Pierre Jourda. Paris: Gallimard, 1956. 661–98.

———. *Propos rustiques.* Edited by Gabriel-André Pérouse and Roger Dubuis. Geneva: Droz, 1994.

Eamon, William. "Cannibalism and Contagion: Framing Syphilis in Counter-Reformation Italy." *Early Science and Medicine* 3, no. 1 (1998): 1–31.

Erasmus. Desiderius. *Colloquies: Collected Works of Erasmus.* Vols. 39 and 40. Translated by Craig R. Thompson. Toronto: The University of Toronto Press, 1997.

———. *Colloquiorum Familiarium formulae.* In the *Opera Omnia Desiderii Erasmi Roterodami,* I–3. Amsterdam: The New Holland Press, 1969.

———. *Erasmi Epistolae.* Vol. 5. Edited by P. S. Allen *et al.* 12 vols. Oxford: Oxford University Press, 1906–1953.

———. *Erasmi Epistolae*. Edited by Craig R. Thompson. Chicago: University of Chicago Press, 1965.

———. *La Correspondance d'Érasme*. Vol. 10. Translated by P. S. Allen, H. M. Allen, and H. W. Garrod. Bruxelles: University Press, 1981.

Fernández Oviedo y Valdes, Gonzalo. *Historia general y natural de las Indias*. Edited by Jose Amador de los Rios. Madrid, 1851.

Fernel, Jean d'Amiens. *Le Meilleur traitement du Mal Vénérien*. 1579. Translated by L. Le Pileur. Paris: G. Masson, 1879.

Fineman, Joel. "The History of the Anecdote: Fiction and Fiction." In *The New Historicism*. Edited by H. Aram Veeser, 49–76. New York: Routledge, 1989.

Fioravanti, Leonardo. *Capricci medicinali*. Venice, 1582.

———. *Della fisica*. Venice, 1582.

———. *Delle specchio di scientie universale*. Venice, 1572.

Foucault, Michel. *Les mots et les choses*. Paris: Gallimard, 1966.

———. *The Order of Things: An Archaeology of the Human Sciences*. A translation of *Les Mots et les choses*. New York: Vintage Books, 1971.

Fracastor, Jérôme. *La Syphilis ou le mal français/Syphilis sive morbus gallicus*. Translated by Jacqueline Vons. Paris: Les Belles Lettres, 2011.

Fragonard, Marie-Madeleine. "Les 'chemins enlacez' des *Tragiques*: *Revue d'Histoire Littéraire de la France*," 92ᵉ Année, N° 4 (July–August 1992): 669–78.

Frisch, Andrea. "In a Sacramental Mode: Jean de Léry's Calvinist Ethnography," *Representations* 77, no. 1 (Winter 2002): 82–106.

———. *The Invention of the Eyewitness: Witnessing and Testimony in Early Modern France*. Chapel Hill: North Carolina Studies in Romance Languages and Literatures, 2004.

Grisoni, Dominique-Antoine. "Sur Jean de Léry. Entretien avec Claude Lévi-Strauss. Propos recueillis par Dominique-Antoine Grisoni." In *Jean de Léry: Histoire d'un voyage faict en la terre de Brésil*. Edited by Frank Lestringant, 5–14. Paris: Le Livre de Poche, 1994.

Guerra, Francesco. "The Problem of Syphilis. " In *First Images of America: The Impact of the New World on the Old*. Edited by Fredi Chiappelli et al., 845–51. 2 vols. Berkeley: University of California Press, 1976.

Harper, Kristin N., Molly K. Zuckerman, and George J. Armelagos. "Syphilis: Then and Now." *The Scientist Magazine*, February 1, 2014, 1–8. http://www.the-scientist.com/TheScientist/daily/2014/02/05a.html.

Harrison, L. W. "The Origin of Syphilis." *British Journal of Venereal Diseases* 35, no. 1 (1959): 1–7.

Healy, Margaret. "Bronzino's London Allegory and the Art of Syphilis." *Oxford Art Journal* 20, no. 1 (1997): 3–11.

Heller, Henry. "Marguerite de Navarre and the Reformers of Meaux." *Bibliothèque d'Humanisme et Renaissance* 33, no. 2 (1971): 271–310.

Henderson, John. *The Renaissance Hospital: Healing the Body and Healing the Soul*. New Haven, CT: Yale University Press, 2006.

Héry, Thierry de. *La Méthode curatoire pour la maladie vénérienne, vulgairement appelée grosse vairolle, et de la diversité des ses symptomes*. Paris: Matthieu David et Arnoud L'Angelier, 1552.

Hirzel, Rudolf. *Der Dialog, Ein Literarhistorischen Versuch*. Leipzig: S. Hirzel, 1895.

Hobart, Brenton. "L'Imaginaire de la peste dans la littérature française de la Renaissance." Thèse de Docteur de l'Université Paris-Sorbonne, 8 janvier 2014.

Holcomb, Richard. "Ruy Diaz de Isla and the Haitian Myth of European Syphilis." *Medical Life* 45 (1956): 270–315.

Huizinga, J. *Erasmus of Rotterdam*. Garden City, New York: Phaidon Publishers, 1952.

Hutten, Ulrich von. *De l'expérience et approbation Ulrich de Hutten notable chevalier touchant la medecine du boys dict guiacum pour circonvenir et deschasser la maladie indeuement appellee françoise. Aincoys par gens de meilleur urgent est dicte et appelee la maladie de Naples traduicte et interpretee par maistre Jehan Cheradame hypocrates estudiant en la faculté et art de medecine*, in-4⁰. Paris: Jean Trepperel, n.d.

———. *Of the Wood Called Guaiacum*. London: Thomas Bertheletreglii, 1540.

———. *Opera omnia*. Edited by Eduard Böcking. Vol. 4. Leipzig, 1859–1870.

Jeanselme, E. *Histoire de la syphilis. Son origine. Son expansion. Progrès realisés dans l'étude de cette maladie depuis la fin du XVe siècle jusqu'à l'époque contemporaine. Extrait du Traité de la syphilis*. Vol. 1. Paris: G. Doin, 1931.

Jillings, Lewis. "The Aggression of the Cured Syphilitic: Ulrich von Hutten's Projections of His Disease as Metaphor." *The German Quarterly* 68, no. 1 (Winter 1995): 1–18.

Knecht, R. J. *The French Wars of Religion 1559–1598*. 2nd ed. London: Longman, 1996.

Kushner, Eva. *Le Dialogue à la Renaissance: Histoire et poétique*. Geneva: Droz, 2004.

———. "Les Colloques et l'inscription de l'autre dans le discours." In *Dix conférences sur Érasme. Éloge de la folie—Colloques*. Edited by Claude Blum, 33–47. Paris/Geneva: Honoré Champion, 1988.

LaCapra, Dominick. *History and Memory After Auschwitz*. Ithaca, NY: Cornell University Press, 1998.

Langer, Ullrich. "A Courtier's Problematic Defense: Ronsard's 'Response aux injures.'" *Bibliothèque d'Humanisme et Renaissance* 46, no. 2 (1984): 343–55.

Léry, Jean de. *Au lendemain de la Saint-Barthélemy. Guerre civile et famine. Histoire mémorable du siège de Sancerre de Jean de Léry*. Edited by Gérald Nakam. Paris: Éditions Anthropos, 1975.

———. *Histoire d'un voyage faict en la terre du Brésil*. 2nd ed. Edited by Frank Lestringrant. Paris: Le Livre de Poche, 1994.

———. *History of a Voyage to the Land of Brazil*. Translated by Janet Whatley. Berkeley: University of California Press, 1992.

Lestringant, Frank. "Catholiques et cannibales. Le thème du cannibalisme ans le discours protestant au temps des guerres de religion." In *Pratiques & Discours alimentaires à la Renaissance. Actes du colloque de Tours 1979*. Edited by J.-C. Margolin et R. Sauzet, 233–45. Paris: Maisonneuve et Larose, 1982.

———. *Le Huguenot et le sauvage. L'Amérique et la controverse coloniale, en France, au temps des guerres de religion*. Geneva: Droz, 2004.

———. *Une sainte horreur ou le voyage en eucharistie*. 2nd ed. Geneva: Droz, 2012.

Leushuis, Reinier. "The Mimesis of Marriage: Dialogue and Intimacy in Erasmus's Matrimonial Writings." *Renaissance Quarterly* 57, no. 4 (Winter 2004): 1278–1307.

Long, Kathleen Perry. "'Child in the Water': The Spectacle of Violence in Théodore Agrippa d'Aubigné's *Les Tragiques*." *Dalhousie French Studies* 8 (Winter 2007): 155–65.

López de Gómara, Francisco. *Histoire générale des Indes occidentales et terres neuves, qui iusques à présent esté descouvertes, augmentée en ceste cinquiesme édition de la descrip-*

tion de la nouvelle Espagne et la grande ville de Mexique, autrement nommé, Tenuctilan, composée en espagnol par François López de Gómara, et traduict en François par S. de Genillé Mart. Fumée. A Paris chez Michel Sonnius, rue sainct Jacques, à l'enseigne de l'escu de Basle, M.D.LXXXVII.

Losse, Deborah N. "The Old World Meets the New in Montaigne's *Essais*: The Nexus of Syphilis, Cannibalism, and Empirical Medicine." *Montaigne Studies* 22, nos. 1–2 (2010): 85–100.

———. "Revisioning Saint Augustine: Rabelaisian Intertexts of Augustine's *Confessions*." *Allegorica* 23 (2002): 19–31.

———. "Rewriting Culture: Montaigne Recounts New World Ethnography." *Neophilologus* 83, no. 4 (1999): 517–28.

———. *Sampling the Book: Reneaissance Prologues and the French Conteurs*. Lewisburg, PA: Bucknell University Press, 1994.

Marchi, Dudley D. "Montaigne and the New World: The Cannibalism of Cultural Production." *Modern Language Studies* 23, no. 4 (Autumn 1993), 35–54.

Maynard, Katherine. "'Miel empoisonné': Satire and Sickness in Ronsard's *Discours des misères de ce temps*." In Renner, *La Satire dans tous ses états*, 245–64.

Ménager, Daniel. *Ronsard: Le roi, le poète et les hommes*. Geneva: Droz, 1979.

Montaiglon, Anatole de. *Recueil de poésies françoises des XVe et XVIe siècles: Morales, facétieuses, historiques*, ed. Anatole de Montaiglon. 3 vols. Paris: P. Jannet, 1855.

Montaigne, Michel de. *The Complete Essays of Montaigne*. Translated by Donald M. Frame. Stanford: Stanford University Press, 1965.

———. *Les Essais*. Edited by Pierre Villey. 3 vols. Paris: Quadrige/Presse Universitaires de France, 1992.

Nakam, Géralde. *Montaigne et son temps: Les événements et les Essais. L'Histoire, la vie et le livre*. Paris: A.-G. Nizet, 1982.

Navarre, Marguerite de. *L'Heptaméron*. Edited by Michel François. Paris: Garnier Frères, 1967.

Pagden, Anthony. *The Fall of Natural Man: The American Indian and the Origins of Comparative Ethnology*. Cambridge: Cambridge University Press, 1986.

Paracelsus. "The *Herbarius* of Paracelsus." Edited by Bruce Moran. *Pharmacy in History* 35 (1993): 99–127.

———. "Herbarius Theophrasti de virtutibus herbarum, radicum seminum etc Alemaniae, patriae et imperii." In *Theophrast von Hohenheim gen. Paracelsus Sämtliche Werke. I. Abteilung:Medizinische, naturwissenschaftliche und philosophische Schriften*. Edited by Karl Sudhoff, vol. 2, 3–58. Munich & Berlin: Oldenbourg, 1930.

Paré, Ambroise. *Dix Livres de la Chirurgie, avec Le Magasin des Instrumens necessaires à icelle*. Paris: Jean le Royer, 1564. Reprint, Paris: Cercle du Livre Précieux, n.d.

———. *Les Oeuvres*. Paris, 1628.

———. *Oeuvres complètes*. Edited by J.-F. Malgaigne. 3 vols. Geneva: Slatkine Reprints, 1970.

Persels, Jeff. "The Sorbonnic Trots: Staging the Intestinal Distress of the Roman Catholic Church in French Reform Theater." *Renaissance Quarterly* 56, no, 4 (Winter 2003): 1089–1111.

Pileur, L. "Gorre et grande gorre." *Bulletin de la Société de l'Histoire de la Médecine* 9 (1910): 217–24.

Popelinière, Henri Lancelot Voisin de la. *L'Histoire de France, enrichie des plus notable occurrances survenues ez provinces de l'Europe et pays voisins, depuis l'an 1550, jusques à ces temps,* par Abraham H, Vol. II, s.1., 1581.

Pot, Olivier. "Prophétie et mélancolie. La querelle entre Ronsard et les protestants (1562–1565)." In *Prophètes et prophéties au XVI^esiècle. Cahiers V-L Saulnier,* 15. 189–229. Paris: Presses de l'ENS, 1998.

Quétel, Claude. *The History of Syphilis.* Translated by Judith Braddock and Brian Pike. Baltimore: Johns Hopkins University Press, 1992.

Rabelais, François. *The Complete Works of François Rabelais.* Translated by Donald M. Frame. Berkeley: University of California Press, 1991.

———. *Oeuvres complètes.* Edited by Guy Demerson. Paris: Éditions du Seuil, 1973.

Renner, Bernd. "From *Satura* to *Satyre:* François Rabelais and the Renaissance Appropriation of Genre." *Renaissance Quarterly* 67, no. 2 (Summer 2014): 377–424.

———, ed. *La Satire dans tous ses états.* Geneva: Droz, 2009.

Rigolot, François. "Poétique et politique: Ronsard et Montaigne devant les troubles de leur temps." In *Ronsard et Montaigne: écrivains engagés?* Edited by Michel Dassonville, 57–69. Lexington, KY: French Forum, 1989.

———."Rabelais, Misogyny, and Christian Charity: Biblical Intertextuality and the Renaissance Crisis of Exemplarity." *PMLA* 109, no. 2 (March 1994): 225–37.

Rodini, Elizabeth. "Functional Jewels." *Art Institute of Chicago Museum Studies* 25, no. 2 (2000): 76–78, 108.

Ronsard, Pierre de. *Oeuvres complètes.* Edited by Gustave Cohen. 2 vols. Paris: Gallimard, 1950.

Silver, Susan K. "'And the Word became Flesh . . .': Cannibalism and Religious Polemic in the Poetry of Desportes and d'Aubigné. " *Renaissance and Reformation/Renaissance et Réforme* 24, no. 1 (2000): 45–56.

Starobinski, Jean. "The Body's Moment." *Yale French Studies* 64 (1983): 273–305.

Szabari, Antonia. *Less Rightly Said: Scandals and Readers in Sixteenth-Century France.* Stanford: Stanford University Press, 2010.

———. "'parler seulement de moy': The Disposition of the Subject in Montaigne's Essay 'De l'art de conferer.'" *MLN* 116, no. 5 (December 2001): 1001–24.

Terpstra, Nicholas. *Lost Girls: Sex and Death in Renaissance Florence.* Baltimore: Johns Hopkins University Press, 2010.

Thevet, André. *Histoire d'André Thevet Angoumousin, cosmographe du Roy, de deux voyages faits aux Indes Australes et Occidentales.* Edited by Jean-Claude Laborie and Frank Lestringant. Geneva: Droz, 2006.

Vicary, Grace Q. "Visual Art as Social Data: The Renaissance Codpiece." *Cultural Anthropology* 4, no. 1 (February 1989), 3–35.

Webster, Charles. "Paracelsus: Medicine as Popular Protest. " In *Medicine and the Reformation.* Edited by Ole Peter Grell and Andrew Cunningham, 57–77. London: Routledge, 1993.

White, Hayden. *Tropics of Discourse: Essays in Cultural Criticism.* Baltimore: Johns Hopkins University Press, 1985.

Williams, George Hunston. *The Radical Reformation.* 3rd ed. Kirksville, MO: Truman State University Press, 2000.

INDEX

Abraham, 53, 127, 128
adultery, 151n17, 152n17; among Guise family, 151n17; in papacy, 152n17
aemulatio, 7. *See also* metaphor
Africa, 1, 27, 139n3
Agesilaus, 15
Ahmed, Ehsan, 4, 130n8
AIDS, 86
Alexander VI, pope, 132n3
Alexandrinus, Johannes, 23
Allen, H. M., 136n12
Allen, P. S., 131n30, 134n20, 136n12
Amboise: Conspiracy of Amboise, 4; Edict of Amboise, 4, 62; Paix d' Amboise, 63
America, 48, 67, 105; American, 75; Americas, viii; South American, vii
Anselme, 55
anthropophagy, 89; *anthropophages*, 9, 57. See also *théophages*
Aphrodite, 60
apothecaries, 147n12
appetite, 117; wild, 76, 111, 143n1; among old women, 76–77
Arabia, 139n3
Arbesmann, Rudolph, 8, 51, 53, 131n22, 134n18, 140n9

Argentier, viii, 6, 86, 96
Aristophanes, 25
Armelagos, George J., 130n3
armies, royal, 73; forces, royal, 108, 109; troops, royal, 125
Asclepiades, 24
Asia, 27
atemporal quality, 84; experience, 80
atheism, 77; atheist, 61, 69, 72, 129n1
Atrée, 151n14
Aubigné, Agrippa d', 2, 5, 6, 7, 8, 10, 63, 105, 106–20, 124, 125, 127, 131n15, 132n32, 133n13, 142n28, 145n13, 149n26, 149n2, 150n5, 150n9, 152n19, 153n5; "Instruction d'Estat," 118–19, 120; "Lettre à la Reine," 118–20, 125, 131n19, 131n31, 132n32, 153n21; *Les Tragiques*, 6, 7, 107–20, 131n15: "La Chambre dorée," 115; "Les Fers," 116; "Les Feux," 116–17; "Jugement," 120, 150n9, 152n17; "Misères," 107–14, 150n5, 150n10, 151n14, 151n15, 151n17; "Vengeances," 114
Augustine, Saint, 8, 51; Augustinian, 9, 24; *Confessions*, 134n23; *le bon pere*, 116
authority: moral, 33
Auxerre, 68

161

INDEX

Averrois, 23
Avignon, 114
Aztecs, 98

Badius, Conrad, 140n8; *Comédie du pape malade et tirant à la fin*, 140n8
Bakhtin, Mikhail, 11, 12, 26, 53, 132n1, 140n11
barbarism, 89
barber, 42
Baudouin, François, 132n33
Beda, Noël, 39
beggars, 55
behavior: lewd or lascivious, 8, 34, 47, 55, 58; social, 35; unnatural, 2, 46, 87, 88; wanton, 26, 35, 40, 118
Bembo, Pietro, 133n8
Bertrand, Dominique, 141n14
Bertulph, 34, 35
Besançon, 12
Bèze, Théodore de, 5, 9, 13, 55, 127, 153n3; *Abraham sacriviant*, 127, 153n6. See also *Satyres chrestiennes de la cuisine papale*
Bible, 52
Bichard-Thomine, Marie-Claude, 141n14
Bierlaire, Franz, 30, 43, 44, 135n1, 136n8, 136n9, 136n10, 137n18, 137n19
Blessus, Pompilius, 40, 137n19
Böcking, Eduard, 133n11
body, 93, 99; corruption, 87, 88; infected, 7 106, 109; the act of becoming, 11; of mother, 109; poisoned, 110; swollen, 110. See also Christ *and* France
body politic, 10, 91, 93, 94, 99, 102, 103, 126; Europe's body and soul, 43; republic as body, 44; social body, 105
Bordeaux: Bordeaux copy (*exemplaire de Bordeaux*), 146n3
Borgia, Cardinal Jean, 132n3
Bourgade, Pierre de la, 82; wife of, 82
Bourges, 55
Boyle, Marguerite O'Rourke, 10, 24, 44, 131n30, 134n20, 138n26, 140n8
Braddock, Judith, 146n5

Brazil (Brésil), 1, 48, 58, 72, 75, 77, 79, 80, 81, 83, 84; Brazilian, 82, 89, 90; Brazil ink, 48, 67, 143n3; indigenous people of, 67, 73, 142n2
breast: bloodied the breast that nourished, 109; breast feeding, 132; breast milk, 37, 38, 39
Briçonnet, Guillaume, 3–4, 63, 130n9
Bronzino, 26
brothels, 39
Brun, Estienne, 16
Brun, Thomas, 137n19
Brunfels, Otto, 97
bubas, las, 32
Bucer, Martin, 133
butcher, 43, 45

Calvin, Jean, 4, 58, 79, 107; *Institutes of the Christian Religion*, 144n6
Calvinist, 4, 125; Calvinist (adj.), 4, 47, 61, 122, 148n19, 149n4; ministers, 49; preachers, 124; concept of witness, 79
cannibalism, vii, viii, 2, 3, 8, 9, 46, 66, 72, 73, 80, 81, 82, 84, 87, 88, 90, 92, 93, 94, 105, 110, 111, 115, 116, 118, 125, 145n13; cannibals, 56, 57, 118; "forced," 75, 76; "violent," 75, 76; moral opposition to, 81; by Christians, 71, 72, 75, 76; narration of, 77, 143n5, 150n11
cardinal, 55, 56
Carthusian, 33–34, 35, 136n8; *chartreux*, 33
Castillon-la-Bataille, 9, 95, 99
Catherine de Medici, 5, 47, 59, 62, 73, 114, 121
Catholicism, 148n19; catholics, 5, 6, 8, 9, 43, 46, 49, 58, 65, 91, 97, 106, 108, 109, 110, 123, 130n12, 132n33, 143n5, 144n7, 149n4; Catholic (adj.), 9, 79, 82; Church, 142n24; clergy, 6, 55, 56, 57; extremists, 7; faith, 5; forces, 6, 78, 82; polemiscists, 141n15; theologians, 63
cause: natural, 8; first cause, 92; root cause, 100. See also prophasis
Cavaillon, H., 139n6

Cavalca, Domenica, 51m 140n9; *Lo Specchio della croce*, 140n9
Cellini, Benvenuto, 132n3
Chamay, Charles-Antoine, 55, 131n26, 141n15
chambre ardente, 4
Champier, Symphorien, 96, 97, 147n16
Chancellor of Poland, 26
chancre, 22, 24, 51; *bosse chancreuse*, 22
Charity, 34, 60, 83; *caritas*, 22
Charles V, 10, 15, 16, 20, 24, 34, 36, 42, 43, 136n9, 138n23
Charles VIII, 3, 32, 136n7
Charles IX, 14, 47, 62
Chiabrena des pucelles, 21
Chiappelli, Fredi, 130
childbirth, 14, 19, 52
children, 33, 34, 36, 41; upbringing of, 31
chinaroot, viii, 91, 96
Chinese, 98
Christ, 4, 23, 24, 43, 44, 51, 83, 90; Christianity, 91; Christians, 14, 71, 141n17; Christian (adj.), 36, 43, 44; Christian principles, 118; Christus medicus, 8, 23, 24, 50, 52, 83, 134n18, 140n8, 140n9; blood of, 5, 49, 53, 117, 144n6; body of, 49, 57, 111, 117, 144n6; glory of, 44
chronicles, 9, 10, 14, 88, 105; chronicler, 2, 68, 82, 85, 121, 123; *Chronique Gargantuine*, 52
Clouet, François, 16, 20
codpiece, 11, 16, 17, 18, 20, 21, 26; backward curve in, 20 22, 29; *braguette*, 15, 16, 17, 22; round, 15; square, 15; absence of, 21
Cohen, Gustave, 62, 131
Coligny, Odet de, cardinal de Châtillon, 23
Colloque of Poissy, 5
colloquy, 5, 31, 32, 34, 42
Columbus, Christopher, viii, 11, 32, 92, 130n3, 144n11
"Complainte de Messire Pierre Liset," 56, 57, 137n20, 153n3
confession: public, 62, 87; confessor, 36

conflict, 123, 124, 125, 127: civic, 9, 34, 55; expanded family, 125; internal, 126; political, 10, 43; religious, 10, 43, 55; world, 36
Conley, Tom, 147n15
contagion, 34
contes/nouvelles, 53
Cooper, Alix, 147n12; 147n16
Cornell, Barbara, 31, 32, 38, 135n2
cosmographer, 1, 6, 46, 73
Cottret, Bernard, 150n11
Counter-Reformation, 88, 98, 141n18
Cowes, William, 3
Crosby, Alfred W., Jr., 104, 105, 149n23, 149n24, 149n25
Crouzet, Denis, 4, 130n10, 149n1, 149n4, 152n20
cruelty, barbarous, 151n12; cruel persecution, 111; cruel transformation, 81, cruel treatment, 78; of Catholics, 64, 82, 83; of Huguenots, 64; of Indigenous peoples of the New World, 89
cuckoldry, 22, 23
cuider (cuyder), 62–63, 79. See also presumption
culture: church, 11; official, 11, popular, 11; cultural practice, 105
Cunningham, Andrew, 147n13
cure, 36: empirical, 105; systemic, 128
customs, 35, 89; English, 35; French, 35; German, 35; Italian, 35; borrowed, 112; corrupted, 114; within cultural context, 69, 89
Cypris, 60. See also Aphrodite

Dante, 100
Dassonville, Michel, 142n23
death: from syphilis, 123; public, 123; slow, 127
Demerson, Guy, 131n24
Désiré, Artus, 5, 9, 58, 106, 122, 131n27, 141n17, 149n1; *Le Contrepoison des cinquante-dix chansons de Clément Marot*, 58–59, 106, 131n27, 141n17, 149n1

De Smet, Ingrid A. R., 132n33, 148n18

Des Périers, Bonaventure, 49, 52, 138n27; *Nouvelles Récréations et joyeux devis*, 138n27

De Thou, Jacques Auguste, 148n18, 152n19; *Hieracosophion*, 148n18, 152n19

Deuteronomy, Book of, 146n17

diagnosis, 8, 86; diagnostic, 101, 102; diagnostician, 86; of melancholy, 142n19

dialogue, 32, 44: familiar, 31; philosophical, 31; dialogical model, 42

Diane de Poitiers, 12, 129n1

Diaz de Isla, Ruy, 85, 105

Diefendorf, Barbara B., 130n12

Dindinault, 28

disease, 2, 7, 9, 10, 11, 12, 14, 18, 23, 29, 30, 44, 86, 92, 105, 121; venereal, 86, 93

disorder, civil, 6, 106

Donahue, Katherine C., 130, 130n3

Don Juan, 32

Douglas, Mary, 93, 146n11

dropsy, 110; dropsied, 111

Droz, Eugénie, 55, 141n15

Dubedout, E. T., 142n25

Dubuis, Roger, 140n14

Du Fail, Noël, 5, 53, 55, 140n13; *Balivernies, ou contes nouveaux d' Eutrapel, autrement dit Léon Ladulphy*, 140n14; *Propos rustiques*, 53, 55, 140n13, 140n14

dyscrasia, 109–10

Eamon, William, 85, 87, 88, 91, 92, 93, 118, 130n4, 130n5, 139n1, 144n11, 145n11, 146n1, 146n2, 146n6, 146n10, 146n11

écolier limousin, 54

Edict of Fontainebleau, 4

Edict of Janvier, 5

Edict of Nantes, 5

Edict of Saint-Germain, 5

Edict of Septembre, 123, 142n27

edicts reculating infected individuals, 50

empiricists, 91, 92; empirical, 100

epic poem, 13

epidemic, 7, 8, 41d, 42, 58, 65, 86, 99; epidemic proportion, 58

Epistemon, 29

epithalamium, 42

Eppendorf, Henri von, 137n19

Erasmus, 2, 4, 5, 10, 13, 24, 26, 27, 29, 30–45, 52, 54, 123, 127, 131n29, 134n20, 135n3, 135n4, 135n6, 136n10, 136n12, 137n15, 137n22, 138n23, 138n24, 140n31; *Colloquies*, 30, 31, 39, 42, 43, 131n29, 135n24: "Coniugium, 42, "The Soldier and the Carthusian, 32–34, 35, 36, 54; "The New Mother," 31, 34, 36–38, 39, 43, 140n4; "Inns," 34–35; "The Young Man and the Harlot, 35–36; "A Marriage in Name Only, 40–42, 135n24; "A Fish Diet," 10, 43–45; "The Praise of Marriage," 42; *Erasmi epistolae*, 131n30, 134n20, 134n22, 138n26, 139n8

Esau, 7, 107, 109, 111

essay, 6, 10

Este, Anne d', 114, 151n17

Estissac, Jean d', 137n15; widow of, 137n15

Estates-General, 120

ethnography, 66; ethnographer, 6, 66, 73. *See also* eye to record accurately

Eucharist, 5, 8, 36, 49, 79, 107, 111, 148n19; eucharistic, 4

Europe, 2, 3, 10, 11, 27, 29, 30, 31, 32, 36, 45, 84, 85, 86, 98, 105, 121, 123, 130

Eutrapelus, 24, 36, 37, 38, 39, 42, 137n15

evangelism, 4; evangelical, 50; evangelical belief, 45; evangelical point of view, 14; evangelical reform, 27, 43; evangelical reformist works, 50

expansion, territorial, 30; New World, 10; of Charles V, 36

experience: in Brazil, 74; of hunger, 74, 109; of illness, 86, 103; medical, 86, 87; over scientific knowledge, 97; of plague, 150n7

explorers, 46, 96, 123

eye of God: heaven's eyes, 116; omniscient, 114
eye to record accurately, 66, 68, 76, 89

Fabulla, 36, 37, 39, 137n15
faith, 2, 3; common, 64; unified, 63; of besieged of Sancerre, 77
family, 5, 27, 36, 39, 45; royal, 26; structure, 31, 42, 45
Fanlo, Jean-Raymond, 107, 110, 120, 131n13, 151n15, 151n17, 152n17, 153n5
farce, 11
fashion: changes in, 12, 15, 17, 19, 20, 29; excesses, 152n19; low, 17
fasting, 44; causing insomnia or delerium, 44
fatherhood, 22; father, absence of, 36
feasting, 44
Fernandez Oviedo y Valdes, Gonzalo, 32, 85, 88, 136n7, 146n2; *Historia general y natural de las Indias*, 146n2
Fernel, Jean, 12, 49, 70, 103, 126, 129n1, 133n5, 139n5, 148n19, 153n4; *Le meilleur traitement du Mal Vénérien*, 129, 133n5, 139n5, 144n10
fertility: decrease in, 26
fever, 14, 88, 104
Fildes, Valerie, 38, 136n13
Fineman, Joel, 8, 131n18
Fioravanti, Leonardo, viii, 2, 6, 86, 87–88, 91–93, 96, 100, 118, 144n11, 148n18; *Capricci medicinali*, 91, 130n5, 146n9; *Della fisica*, 146n10
fishmonger, 43, 45
Florence, 99, 124, 137n14
forces: English, 126, foreign, 126, Spanish, 126
fornication, 151n17
Foucault, Michel, 7, 131n16, 131n17
Fracastor, Jérôme, 129n1, 133n8; Fracastorius, Hieronymus, 138n25; Fracastoro, Girolamo, 3, 133n8, 133, 138n25; *La Syphilis ou le mal français/Syphilis sive morbus gallicus*, 3, 8, 13, 129
Fragonard, Marie-Madeleine, 152n17

Frame, Donald, 129n1, 131n14, 133n6
France, viii, 2, 3, 6, 9, 10, 24, 30, 43, 62, 64, 99, 120, 121, 124; infected body of, 1, 101; King of France, 43; Mother France, 107, 109, 11, suffering mother, 7, 109; survival of, 128; weakened, 119, 128; the French, 64, 107, 123, 125; French invasion of Italy, 11, 32, 100, 102, 105, 112, 123, 124, 125, 127
François I, 4, 10, 15, 20, 34, 36, 43, 44, 125, 132n3, 134n17, 136n9, 138n23
François II, 4, 47
freedom: of conscience, 78, 84; of worship, 5
French disease, 105, 136n7
friendship, 41; *amicitia*, 41; *phila*, 41
Frisch, Andrea, 79–80, 106, 143n6, 145n16, 149n4
Fuchs, Remacle, 3

Gabriel, 40, 41, 42
Galen, 24
Gargamelle, 19, 38, 39, 75
Gargantua, 14, 19, 20, 27, 29, 38, 39, 41, 155n24
Garrod, H. W., 136n12
Geneva, 9, 47, 60; theologians of, 65
Germany, 30
Ghibelline, 99
Gilbert, Judson B., 134n17
"God of white dough," 57
gorre des marranes, 3, 130n6
Gospel, 61; l'Évangile, 61
Goulart, Simon, 149n4
goutteux, 5, 9, 11, 12, 24, 25; gout, 53, 140n11
grace, God's, 79; scorn of, 83
Grandgousier, 19, 137n23
Gregory XV, Pope, 153n5
Grell, Ole Peter, 147n18
grill (*boucan*), 67
Grisoni, Dominique-Antoine, 143n2
grotesque, 11

INDEX

Grünpeck, Joseph, 3
guaiacum (*gayac*), vii, 91, 96, 133n11, 141n18
Guelph, 99
Guerra, Francesco, 1, 130n3, 139n3, 144n8
Guise: family, 149n4, 151n15; François, duc de, 151n17

habits, 87; continuity in, 88, 92, 96, 103; dietary, 104; respect for, 104
Harper, Kristin N., 130n3
Harrison, L. W., 54, 133n4, 139n3, 139n6
health, 24, 25, 26, 41, 42, 52; individual, 99, 105; of body politic, 99; of France, 63, 120; of mind and body, 44, 105; *santé*, 25, 26, 52, 131n24
Healy, Margaret, 26, 27, 134n21, 134n22
Heller, Henry, 4, 130n8
Henderson, John, 8, 9, 51, 131n21, 140n9, 141n18
Henri II, 4, 12, 14, 25, 126, 129n1
Henri III, 14, 47, 99, 107, 115, 126, 139n7, 150n5; "degenere Henry," 115
Henri de Navarre, 118, 126, 150n5; Henri IV, 118, 150n5; Henri le grand, 127
Henry VIII, 16, 20, 24, 44, 131n30, 134n17, 140n8
heresy, 9, 58, 106; heretics, 118, 136n11: Protestant, 4; Reformist, 122
Héry, Thierry de, 130n7
Hippocrates, 23
Hirzel, Rudolf, 32, 135n5
Hobart, Brenton, 104, 148n18, 150n7, 150n9
Holbein, Hans, the Younger, 16, 20
Holcomb, Richard, 146n2
Holy Spirit, 79, 81, 107
Homer, 148n18
host, 8, 57, 144n6; Calvinist view of, 150n9
Huguenot(s), 4, 5, 6, 59, 106–7, 122, 123, 125, 127, 128, 139n4, 143n5, 145n13, 150n4; besieged, 77, 78;

Huguenot (adj.), 9; cause, 78; ministers, 83; pamphleteers, 120; preacher, 60, 61, 62; theology, 59
Huizinga, J., 135n1
hunger, 36, 109; expertise on, 74, 77; iconic image of, 74; moral effect of, 81, 113; narrative of, 75; phenomenon of hunger, 73, 109, psychology of famine, 80; starvation, 108, 116, 128
Hutten, Ulrich von, 14, 15, 105, 132n3, 133n9, 133n11, 137n19, 149n24, 149n25
hygiene: changes in, 29n31; communal, 42; lack of hygiene in inns, 34, 42
hypocrisy: Hugenot, 142n24; hypocrite, 60, 127

imagination, viii, 10, 66, 88
imitator, great, 139n3. *See also* syphilis
Incas, 98
incest, 151n17; incestuous, 114
incurabili, 9; hospitals for, 141n18
infanticide: maternal struggle with, 113
infection, 9, 65; infected, 105; infects, 119; festering smell, 116
inhumanity, 97; towards inhabitants of New World, 97–98
intolerance, 93, 125
invention, 74, 78, 109; inventive spirit, 74
Iphigenia, 40, 41
irony, 32
Isaac, 127
Iswolsky, Hélène, 132n1
Italy, 2, 12, 30, 32, 53, 86, 136n7; French invasion of, 92

Jacob, 7, 107, 109, 111
Jan, frère, 28, 29
Jean d' Albret, 127
Jeanselme, E., 32, 132n2, 132n3
Jews, 98, 117
Jillings, Lewis, 14, 133n9
Johanneau (*Bailif*), 82; widow Johanneau, 82

INDEX   167

joints, pain in, 33, 40, 53, 100, 106, 122, 153n2

Kasprzyk, Krystyna, 138n27
Kertsner, David, 132n2
kidney stones, 6, 93; as inherited illness, 87
Knecht, R. J., 130n11
knight, 31, 40, 41
knowledge, scientific, 86, 103
Kramer, Kyra Cornelius, 134n17
Kushner, Eva, 32, 33, 135n4, 135n5

Laborie, Jean-Claude, 129n1
Labriolle, Pieere de, 134n23
LaCapra, Dominick, 107–8, 150n6
La Châtre, Claude de, 77–79, 82; request for Léry's account of the siege, 78, 108
Langer, Ullrich, 64, 123, 142n26, 142n27
La Roche-Chandieu, Antoine de, 61, 142n21
Las Casas, Bartolomé de, 85, 88, 146n2; *Historia de las Indias*, 146n2
laughter: community of, 57; of carnival, 53
law: dietary, 44; natural as distinct from unnatural, 88; rule of, 101, 112; disrespect for 112; lawlessness, 117, of the monarch, 64
lechery, 8, 48, 144n8. See also *paillardise*
Lefèvre d' Étaples, Jacques, 4
legno santo, 91. See also guiacum
leprosy, 40; leper's blood, 85
Léry, Jean de, 2, 3, 5, 6, 8, 9, 47, 48, 56, 57, 66–84, 88, 89, 108, 109, 110, 111, 113, 114, 121, 125, 130n2, 131n25, 133n11, 145n13, 145n16; cross-references between works, 73, 75, 84; moralist, 70, 108; Lery-oussou, 71; *Histoire d' un voyage faict en la terre de Brésil*, 48–49, 66, 68, 69, 70, 71, 73, 75, 76, 79, 80, 81, 82, 88, 108, 115, 130n2, 131n25, 139n4, 145n12, 145n17, 146n17, 146n18; *Histoire mémorable du siège de Sancerre*, 6, 67, 68, 71, 73–84, 108, 125, 145n17, 146n17, 150n8, 150n11

Lestringant, Frank, 63, 76, 81, 84, 90, 109, 111, 130n2, 139n4, 141n16, 143n3, 143n5, 144n7, 148n18, 148n19, 149n2 150n11, 151n14, 153n2
Leushuis, Renier, 41, 135n4, 137n22
Lévi-Strauss-Claude, 66, 68, 143n2
Life of Saint Margaret, 14, 52
Ligue (la), 7, 99, 114
likeness, 7
livery, 15, 17, 19, 21; clothing, 29
Lizet, Pierre, 13, 55, 56, 123, 141n15; *Adversum pseudo-evangelicam haeresim*, 13
Long, Kathleen Perry, 149n2
Lopez de Gomara, Francisco, 5, 130n13; *Historia general de las Indias*, 5, 130n13
Lorraine, cardinal de, 114, 115, 151n17; sodomite, 114; incestuous defiler, 114
Losse, Deborah N., 13, 131n17, 133n11, 134n23, 139n1, 139n7, 143n4, 146n7, 147n15
Louis XII, 139n7
Louis XIII, 120, 126, 127
Louise de Savoie, 4
lower stratum ("bas corporel"), 12, 53
Lucretia, 35, 36, 136n11
lues venerea, 3, 129n1; *lues* (disease), 86
Luke, Saint, 23, 24, 53
Luther, Martin, 58
Lyon, 12, 67, 68

mal de Naples (le), 1, 53; *morbus neapolitanus*, 3
mal français (le), 12
mal francese, 35
mala de Franzos, 3
Man of Sorrows, 8. See also Santa Maria Nuova
Marchi, Dudley D., 89, 146n8
Margolin, J.-C., 141n16
Marguerite de Navarre, 3, 4, 41, 52, 63, 136n11; Duchess of Alençon, 3; Mar-

INDEX

guerite d' Angoulême, 130n9; *Heptaméron*, 136n11

Marguerite de Valois, 115

Marie de Medici, 8, 10, 118, 119, 120, 125, 126

Marot, Clément, 58; *Cinquante deux psalmes de David*, 141n17; French translation of Psalms of David, 58

marriage, 5, 22, 36; annulment of, 41; bride, 40; bridegroom, 40; choice of spouse, 27; clandestine, 135; injustice of, 40; structure, 41; responsibility of parents, 41; title-seeking, 40, 42

martyr, 118, 127; martyrdom, 82; martyred child, 111

Mass, 50, 63, 112, 124, 151n16

massacre, 128, *de la Saint-Barthélemy*, 127, des Innocents, 127, de Vassy, 5

Maynard, Katherine, 141n19

medical discourse, 89, 95, 100

medical doctors, 90, 97; Hippocratic, 8; empirical, 92; folk practitioners, 92, 95, 96; physicians, 9, 12, 23, 29, 31, 32, 38, 46, 48, 50, 51, 86, 87, 91, 92; first physicians, 92

medical observation, 93

medical opinion, 108

Medici family, 124, 125

medicine, 6, 8, 86, 97, 125: Arabic, 147n42; empirical, 92, 95; natural, 92; scientific, 87, 92, 96; changes in, 87; practice of, 6, 86, 91

memories, 107; memoirs, 107; reflections, 107

Ménager, Daniel, 142n25

mercenaries, 7, 21, 32, 34, 53, 54, 90, 112; German, 110

mercury: ointment, 14, 17

metaphor, 2, 7, 8, 34, 121, 106; medical metaphor, 93, 99, 138n24; new, 121; prefatory, 131n17

Mexico, 97; Mexicans, 98

Millanges, Simon, 148n18

missionaries, 46, 73, 123

moderation, 10, 25, 44, 99

monarchs, 34, 63; benevolent, 114; providers of France, 114

monk, 54, 55

Montaiglon, Anatole de, 50, 53, 131n23, 139n7, 140n12

Montaigne, Michel de, vii, viii, 2, 5, 6, 7, 8, 63, 68, 71, 73, 85–105, 106, 108, 148n19, 150n7, 152n19; *Les Essais*, 38, 67, 80, 106,112, 120, 123, 124, 125, 127, 129n1, 131n14, 132n33, 137n15, 146n3, 148n18: "De l' art de conférer," 86; "Des cannibales," 89, 90, 94, 143n4; "Des coches," 97–98; "De l' expérience," 86, 88, 101–4; "Des lois sumptuaires," 152n19; "De la phisionomie," 99–101, 112, 123, 125, 132n33; "De la ressemblance des enfans aux peres," 94–96; *Journal de voyage*, 148n19; Pierre Eyquem, 147n15

Montcaret, 99

Montmorency, duc de, 118, 119, 120

morality: conviction, 98; courage, 98, efforts; 98, moral rudder, 101; corrupt morals, 115

Moran, Bruce, 147n12

morbus gallicus, 1, 3, 12, 53, 85

mother, 35; new mother, 37, risks to, 31

Nakam, Géralde, 68, 70, 99, 109, 112, 143n1, 145n14, 145n15, 147n17, 151n13

Naples, 1, 3,32, 85, 91. *See also* mal de Naples

narrator, 19, 21, 22, 24, 81, 84

nature, law of, 44; source of strength in childbirth, 37, to nurse newborn, 37

natural remedies, 91; herbal, 92; efficacy of in New World, 94; local provenance, 97

negotiation, 126

Neuchâtel, 4

New Testament, 136n10, 136n11

New World, 2, 9, 11, 32, 85, 88, 90, 91, 105, 126; exploration, 2, 93; indigenous people of, 49, 58, 65, 73, 91,92,

98, 123, 130n3, 138n25; indigenous women, 1
Niçaise, messire, 56
nursing a child: benefits of, 37; familiar nourishment, 37, 38; ingest mother's mental and physical traits, 38

obsidional cannibalism, 150n11
ointment, therapeutic, 13, 14, 16, 17, 51, 52
Old Testament, 80, 84
Old World, vii, viii, 6, 46, 49, 65, 90, 92, 105, 144n11
Ouetaca, 9, 49
"oubliance," 149n2

Pagden, Anthony, 2, 88, 130n4, 139n1, 145n11, 146n6
paillardise, 1, 9, 47, 48, 55, 58, 115; *paillardé*, 69, 72, 144n7. See also lechery
pandemic, 10, 11, 30, 91, 123; language of, 93; new, 121
Pantagruel, 15, 21, 22, 27, 28, 29, 55
Pantagruélisme, 24
Panurge, 15, 16, 17, 18, 20, 21, 22, 26, 27, 28, 29, 55, 134n16, 134n23, 140n13
Paracelsus, viii, 6, 86, 96, 147n12; Von Hohenheim, Theophrast, 147n12; *Herbarius*, 147n12
Paré, Ambroise, 14, 17, 103, 121, 133n10, 144n9, 147n13, 148n18, 148n21, 153n2
Parlement de Paris, 4; parlements, 4, *arrêt de Parlement de Paris*, 12, 54; *président*, 13, 55
Paris, 8, 12; Parisians, 17, 18; "haulte dame de Paris," 18, 134n16; walls of Paris, 15
Parlamente, 41
Paschal, Pierre de, 148n22
"Patenostre des Verollez," 9, 50–52; Pater Noster, 50, 51
patient, 14, 23, 86, 87, 92, 103, 104; long-suffering, 6, 96
Paul, Saint, 51, 59

Pavia, 138n23
peace, 30, 43, 63, 106, 118, 128
people, of the world, 43–44; indigenous, 46; innocent, 62; united, 107
Périgordin, 110, 11
Pérouse, Gabriel-André, 140n14
persecution, 116, 117
Persels, Jeff, 106, 122, 140n8, 149n3
Peru, 97
pestilence, 10, 44, 125, 148n18; pestilential, 126
Petrarch, 100
Petronius, 40, 42
pians, maladie de, 1, 47, 48, 49, 130n2, 144n8
Pike, Brian, 146n5
Pileur, L., 130n6
pilgrim, 22; pilgrimage, 55; pilgrimage to Rome, 36
Pineaux, Jacques, 122, 153n1
Pine-Coffin, R. S., 134n23
pinta, 1, 139n3
plague, 18, 19, 40, 41–42, 100, 108, 148n18, 150n7
Plato, 23, 86
Poissy, colloque de, 136n33
pollutions, 88, 91
pomander: *pomme d' ambre*, 17, 18; *pomme d' orange*, 17, 18
pope, 43, 55, 56, 125; papacy, 151n17; papal banquet, 57; papal kitchen, 57; papists, 49
Popelinière, Henri Lancelot Voisin de la, 149n1
Portuguese, 89, 98
postules, 9, 17, 48, 88, 118; sore as metaphor, 131; syphilitic sores, 43, 106, 130n5
Pot, Olivier, 141n19
Potard family, 71, 72, 75, 81, 151n12; conversion to Catholicism, 77; profligacy of, 77; weakness of, 77
pox, viii, 1, 2, 8, 15, 22, 23, 24, 29, 32, 33,

34, 36, 42, 45, 50, 53, 60, 62, 129; French, 32, 33; poxied, 5, 41; poxy, 13; rhetoric of, 9, 59, 128; Spanish, 32, 35; spread of, 36, 39

presumption, 62–63, 79, 98. See also *cuider/cuyder*

Priapus, 25

priest, 55, 56, 60

prognosis, 8

prostitution, 36

Protestantism, 91; Protestant, 5, 8, 9, 43, 46, 50, 58, 65, 73, 98, 99, 106, 108, 109, 110, 122–23, 127, 130n12, 132n33, 142n27, 144n7; Protestant (adj.), 14, 125, 127, 151n16: minister, 60; religion, 61

purge: violent, 2, 87–88

quarantine, 41

Queen Mother: Catherine de Medici, 63, 115; Marie de Medici, 118, 119, 120, 125, 126

Quétel, Claude, 100, 146n5

Rabelais, François, 2, 4, 5, 9, 10, 11–29, 38, 41, 49, 52–53, 54, 63, 75, 123, 131n24, 132n1, 133n6, 136n12, 144n8; *Gargantua*, 11, 19–22, 38–39, 75, 133n12, 137n16, 137n17; *Pantagruel*, 11–19, 52, 133n12, 140n10; *Le Quart Livre*, 23–28, 52–53, 131n24; *Le Tiers Livre*, 19, 21–23, 27, 55, 135n24, 137n21, 144n8

reason, natural, 63

recycling imagery, 76

redemption, 51

Reformation, 100

Reform, 118, 153n1: ideology, 127; Reformed: Church, 47, 48, 58, 77; Christians, 69; ministers 47; pamphlets, 75; preachers, 59. See also evangelical reform

religion: "ceux de la religion," 78, 80, 83; religious: conflict, 7; controversy, 3, 31, 58; practices, 121

remedies, 106, 126, 133n8; bitter, 95; common, 119; exotic, 91, 96; preventative, 101; topical, 128. See also natural remedies

Renner, Bernd, 133n12, 139n7, 141n15, 141n19

resemblance, 7; Calvinist antipathy for, 144n6. See also likeness

rhetoric, 63, 122: of medicine, 85; of Catholic polemicists, 59; of Reformed polemicists, 59; rhetorical: paradox, 5; parody, 5. See also pox, rhetoric of

rhubarb, 120

Rigolot, François, 134n16, 142n23

ritual: of Tupinamba ceremony, 68, 89

Robel, Andrée, 132n1

Roche-Chandieu, Antoine de la, 60, 62

Rodini, Elizabeth, 18, 134n15

Roesslin, Eucharias, 136n13

Rolandine, 41

Rome, 119, 124

Ronsard, Pierre de, 5, 9, 59–65, 83, 87, 93, 124, 125, 131n28, 142n19, 142n20, 142n23, 142n24, 142n25, 148n22; "Continuation du discours des miseres de ce temps," 59, 93; "Response de Pierre de Ronsard aux injures et calomnies de je ne sçay quels predicantereaux et minestreaux de Genève," 9, 59–65, 83, 87, 142n21, 142n22

Rouen, 49

sacrements: literal interpretation, 5; symbolic, 5

sailors, 11; Columbus's crew, 32, 53, 92, 144n11

Saint Bartholomew Massacre, 8, 130n12, 149n4, 152n20. See also *massacre de la Saint-Barthélemy*

Sainte-Foy-la-Grande, 99

Sancerre, 6, 67, 72, 77, 80, 125; besieged of, 73, 77, 146n17; siege of, 6, 73–84; surrender of, 6

Saint Pierre, Monsieur de, 78

Saint-Victor, Abbé de, 13. See also Lizet, Pierre

salvation, 44, 53

Santa Maria Nuova, 140n9

Sarrieu, maître de camp, 78, 79

sarsaparilla, vii, 88, 91, 96

satire, 15; Ciceronian, 31, 32; Juvenal and, 31; Lucianic satire, 31, 42, 135n4; satirical narrative, 5; satirical verse, 5, 50, 55

Satyre chrestienne de la cuisine papale, 9, 13, 131n26, 132n7, 133n7, 141n15, 153n3. See also Théodore de Bèze

Sauzet, R. S., 141n16

Scaliger, 103, 148n19

Scythians, 67, 89

self-citation, 79, 80, 84, 146n17

self-effacement, 83

self-portraiture, 6

Sept marchans de Naples, 53–54

Serpon, Minister, 116; daughter of, 116, 153n20

sexual relations, 12, 34, 41, 42, 46, 47; sexual intercourse, 12, 29; sexual mores, 21; sexual pleasure, 12; sexual prowess, 29; avoidance of sexual liaisos with Tupi women by French, 70; unhealthy sexual acts, 115

Siberia, 139n3

sickness, 58, 85, 136n7; global, 65; *implicite*, 119, 125; metaphor of, 93, 101; moral, 65; motion, 97; physical, 7; self-inflicted, 105; spiritual, 106; sick: individual, 101; kingdom, 65, 101, 120; sickroom, 7, 120, 125

siege literature, 6, 100

Silver, Susan K., 145n13

simile, 7

Socrates, 102; Socratic voice, 135n4

sodomy, 152n17

soldiers, 31, 32, 34, 36, 125, 136n8; French, 12, 136n7; German, 11, 21, 32; Italian, 11, 21, 136n7; Spanish, 11, 136n7, 138n26; Swiss, 11; itinerant lives of, 33

Sophronius, 35, 36

Sorbonne: professors, 13, 53, 55; theologians, 39

Soulié, Marguerite, 153n6

Spain, 3, 119; Spaniards, 85; Spanish, 98, 125

spectators, 107, 120

Starobinski, Jean, 95, 100, 101, 147n13, 148n20, 148n21

Sudhoff, Karl, 147n12

suicide (*autochryre*), 110

surgeon, 2, 31, 38, 42, 46, 48, 51, 88, 121, 122

Switzerland, 30

Sypher, G. Wylie, 141n18

symptoms, 7, 12, 13; physical, 34; of civil war, 100, 104; of syphilis, 40, 52, 53, 122; symptomatic, 141n18

Syphile, 3, 13, 129

syphilis, viii, 1, 3, 5, 9, 29, 32, 34, 50, 53, 55, 66, 86, 90, 92, 93, 118, 126, 137n14, 139n3; endemic syphilis, 1; venereal syphilis, 1; syphilitics, 13, 14, 24, 51; epidemic of, 6; as metaphor, 8, 30, 91, 93, 100, 104; outbreak of, 2, 10, 30, 32, 46, 88, 127; prevention of, 42; progression of, 100; spread of, viii, 1, 26, 29, 30, 31, 53, 121; treatment of, 18, 88, 96, 106; transmission of to wives and children, 38, 48. See also symptoms

Szabari, Antonia, 57, 59, 61–62, 86–87, 135n4, 142n23, 146n4

Tailleboudin, 55, 140n13

Terpstra, Nicholas, 38, 137n14

testimony, 32, 111; efficacious testimony, 107; spiritual testimony, 79

Thaumaste, maistre, 17, 18, 26

theology, 8, 107; theologians, 46, 53; reform-minded, 13

théophages, 9, 57. See also *anthropophages*

Thevet, André, 1, 2, 3, 46, 47, 48, 56, 58, 65, 67, 73, 82, 88, 121, 129n1, 139n2; *Cosmographie universelle*, 47, 48, 73; *Histoire de deux voyages*, 46, 47, 129n1, 144n8; *Les Singularitez de la France antarctique*, 47, 73, 88

Thompson, Craig R., 34, 131n29

Thucydides, 148n18

Thyeste, 151n14

Tiberius, 102

Tiraqueau, André, 24, 25

Titian, 16, 20

Torella, Gasparis, 132n2

transubstantiation, 63, 111; Catholic concept of, 9, 49, 57; literal, satirical interpretation, 57; Huguenot interpretation, 117, 150n9

travel literature, 6

treatment, medical, 14, 29, 86; changes in, 12, 29, 96, 103; herbal, 14; thermal baths, 95, 96, 97; violent therapies, 87, 92

tripe, 74, 75

treponema pallidum: subspecies pallidum (syphilis), 144n8; subspecies pertenue, 144n8; subspecies endemicum (bejel), 130n3

truchemens, 69, 70, 72; Norman interpreter, 49, 69, 77, 115

Turner, L. H., 139n3

Tupinamba, 2, 57, 67, 69, 70, 72, 89, 90, 98, 144n8; Tupi, 48, 57, 70, 71; women, 68, 143n5

ulcer, 43, 104, 132n32

Valois, 139n7

Veeser, H. Aram, 131n18

vengeance: extreme, 67, 89, 93; against enemies, 67, 76; Tupi act of, 57

vérole, 1, 23, 47, 55, 60, 86, 123; *vérolé/vérolez*, 5, 9, 11, 12, 52, 132n3, 140n11; *grande vérole*, 3; *grosse vérole (grosse vairolle)*, 3, 12, 50; *petite vérole*, 48, 148n18

Verstegan, Richard, 153n2

Vicary, Grace Q., 16 17, 18, 20, 21, 134n14, 134n17

Villegagnon, Nicolas de, 47, 49, 57, 69–70, 82, 83

Villey, Pierre, 129n1, 131n14

Virgil, 148n18

Voisin de la Popelinière, Henri Lancelot, 149n1

Vons, Jacqueline, 3, 129n1, 130n6

Wars of Religion, viii, 2, 3, 5, 8, 47, 48, 66, 93, 97, 99, 100, 106, 125, 127, 130, 148n18, 148n22

Webster, Charles, 147n12

wet nurse, 12, 34, 132; risks for newborn, 31, 34, 37; opting for, 37, risks to nurse, 38

Whatley, Janet, 84, 1393

White, Hayden, 8, 121, 131n20

will of God, 44, 51, 52

William, 34, 35

Williams, George Hunston, 136n11

witness, 32, 73, 78, 79–80, 81, 107; witnessing, 106; eye witness, 110, 111

Wurtz, Felix, 136n13

yaws, 1, 139n3, 144n8

Zaccheus, 52–53

Zamariel (frère), 60, 61, 62, 63, 64, 83; Huguenot detractor, 125

Zuckerman, Molly K., 130n3

www.ingramcontent.com/pod-product-compliance
Lightning Source LLC
Chambersburg PA
CBHW020948230426
43666CB00005B/232